PRAISE FOR
Stress Solutions for Pregnant Moms

"Dr. Susan Andrews has created an indispensable handbook for every mother-to-be. Drawing on the latest research about high stress during pregnancy and how it can impact a child's development, she offers timely, practical, and empowering solutions. Her easy-to-use guide shows step by step how to effectively manage stress and anxiety during pregnancy. This excellent book will help you and your baby achieve your maximum potential. I highly recommend it."

—DANIEL G. AMEN, MD, author of *Change Your Brain, Change Your Life* and *Healing ADD*

"Be at ease, Susan Andrews shows us why knowing about stress is an essential key in creating harmony and health during a mother's journey. She provides tips and exercises with the breath, listening, and movement that will improve your day. Whether you are a professional, a family member, a mother-to-be or just a friend, take this book and listen deeply to the wisdom that easily helps us tune in and tune up."

—DON CAMPBELL, author of *The Mozart Effect* and *Healing at the Speed of Sound*

"In her neuropsychology practice, Dr. Susan Andrews goes the extra mile in providing both assessment of difficulties and solutions to these problems for her patients. With this book, she describes a global problem—the impact of stress on pregnant women and their unborn children. Then she creates a baseline stress level assessment tool and strategies for stress reduction that have universal value, whether you are a pregnant mom or not. Her well-researched book gives pregnant moms and others who will listen a head start in reducing stress personally, professionally, and in relationships."

—BILLIE M. THOMPSON, PH

"An extremely valuable contribution to one of the most critical issues of our time. *Stress Solutions for Pregnant Moms* offers a wonderful new approach to caring for and honoring yourself and your child during the delicate and formative months of pregnancy. For as you'll find out in this wise and practical book, what you do while you are pregnant can affect your child for years to come."

—PATRICIA SPADARO, author of *Honor Yourself: The Inner Art of Giving and Receiving*

"Even though I have practiced medicine for over 35 years, I learned something new and valuable as I read *Stress Solutions for Pregnant Moms*. Now I have included a discussion of stress management into my prenatal discussion with the patient and her husband. *Stress Solutions for Pregnant Moms* is a well written and important book for pregnant women."

—JOHN HEVRON, MD, OB/GYN

"A treasure trove of information, guidelines, and solutions for coping with and counteracting the effects of stress in our lives. This book is beneficial not only for pregnant women but for anyone. Dr. Andrews has come up with a formula that empowers us to control the effects of stress in our lives and that puts every individual on the path of wellness."

—PATRICIA H. ARNAZZI, MD, Tormed Women's Medical Group

STRESS SOLUTIONS

for

PREGNANT
MOMS

STRESS SOLUTIONS
for
PREGNANT
MOMS

How Breaking Free from Stress Can Boost Your Baby's Potential

Susan Andrews, PhD

TIME SPAN PRESS
Hillsboro, OR
Member of Washington County
COOPERATIVE LIBRARY SERVICES

For information, address:

Twin Span Press
2626 N. Arnoult Rd., Ste. 220
Metairie, Louisiana 70002

E-mail: sandrews@twinspanpress.com

For foreign and translation rights, contact Nigel J. Yorwerth
E-mail: nigel@PublishingCoaches.com

Library of Congress Control Number: 2011937752

ISBN: 978-0-9838984-0-5 5039 0029 12/12

10 9 8 7 6 5 4 3 2 1

Cover design: Nita Ybarra
Interior design: Becky Sheehan

In memory of my mom . . .
and to future generations of mothers
and daughters and their children

Contents

Acknowledgments

MY SINCERE APPRECIATION goes to colleagues, friends, and family who have encouraged me to follow my dream of bringing this information into sharper perspective in the world. Randee Booksh, Billie Thompson, Janet Sweeney, and Melissa Aubert read earlier drafts and provided important feedback.

Alfred Tomatis, Bernard Auriol, Kirk Thompson, Francoise Nicoloff, Dorinne Davis, Paul Madaule, Suzanne Morris, Len Young, and Alex Doman are among the many colleagues who contributed to the Stress Solutions Resource Guide. Thank you.

I owe much gratitude to Don Campbell, who I think of as a mentor and friend. Don has given his time and advice freely.

My profound appreciation goes to my patient and gifted editor, Patricia Spadaro, and to Nigel Yorwerth of Yorwerth Associates/PublishingCoaches.com. Thank you, Patricia and Nigel, for all your vision, support, and expertise in helping me shape this work.

I know my mom would have been so proud of me had she lived to see the final copy. A special thank you goes to my grandson, Colin, and to his parents, Buffy Andrews and Christopher Berry. Colin and his mother truly embody what a baby born to a mom who watched her stress levels during pregnancy is like. My son, Scott Andrews, is always there for me and he is the one who asks those questions that somehow help clarify my thoughts.

Finally, my deep appreciation and love to Michelle, who bolstered my confidence when it flagged and offered suggestions that improved the final product.

PART ONE

*Stress and
Your Pregnancy*

1

An Ounce of Prevention

Prevention is better than cure.
—Desiderius Erasmus

Over the years, researchers have discovered many factors
that can, for better or worse, affect babies during the delicate
first nine months of their lives in the womb. With each
discovery, pregnant women all over the world have complied
by watching what they eat, avoiding alcohol and smoking,
and letting someone else clean the cat box. Yet despite doing
"all the right things," childhood problems with attention,
learning, and anxiety are on the rise—dramatically. What
have we overlooked that may be contributing to the rise of
these problems?

As a child neuropsychologist, I have evaluated and treated
hundreds of children with many types of learning and developmental problems. I have also worked with many parents
who were worried about their children's future. In my search
for new and more effective tools to boost children's learning potential and treat childhood disorders, I found studies
that pointed to an alarming rise in anxiety-related problems
among both children and adults. It seemed logical that there
might be a connection between the rise in anxiety among

adults and the increase in anxiety among children. After digging further into this question, I discovered an astonishing link between anxious pregnant women and many behavioral and emotional problems that show up in their children.

Medical historians long ago identified that war and natural disasters have significant effects on the children born to women who were pregnant during those events. As it turns out, though, the trauma of a single catastrophic ordeal is not the only kind of stress that can potentially affect an unborn child. A mounting body of evidence clearly links sustained high levels of stress and anxiety during pregnancy to many of today's major issues of birth and childhood, such as low birth weight and preterm birth, difficulty coping in emotional situations, learning disabilities, attention deficit, and childhood anxiety.

A wealth of research about the effects of prenatal stress—stress experienced during pregnancy—has been emerging over the past 40 years. In scientific terms, this body of knowledge is brand new and is just starting to reach the general public. While more research still needs to be done, what we have learned already is so vital to the health of future generations that I knew I had to write a book on this one key issue—the potential dangers that too much stress can pose for pregnant women and their babies—so that mothers-to-be and those who support them could immediately begin to understand and integrate this new information into their daily lives.

Simply put, I believe the information in this book is *equal to—if not more important than—the well-recognized warnings for expecting mothers to avoid alcohol and stop smoking.* Yes, dealing effectively with stress, especially while you are pregnant, is that crucial to you, your baby, and our future.

Managing Your Stress
Will Benefit You and Your Baby

Not all stress, of course, is bad. Stress can be thought of as a continuum ranging from having positive effects on us to having very negative effects. On the positive end of this continuum are events that stimulate us and cause us to adjust our behavior and to think and stretch and grow. On the negative end are the kinds of aggravations that make us worry, feel tense and nervous, or feel as if we are always under attack.

Events on the stimulating end of the continuum are often good for us and may be good for a developing baby. And, under normal circumstances, a healthy body and a normal nervous system will naturally reduce the effects of stress, even some of the more negative ones, once the stressful events are over. The problem arises when life's daily stressful events pile up *and* we fail to recognize that our body is not automatically reducing the chemical byproducts building up in our body and brain as a result of trying to cope with those events. In other words, it's not the events themselves that can cause the damage but what happens in our mind and body as a result of the events.

Obviously, stress-producing events are potentially everywhere and it is impossible to avoid them. So I'm not going to tell you to avoid stress. That would be unrealistic. Stress is a part of everyone's life and you can take steps to effectively deal with it. Instead of writing a book warning of dangers and heaping more worry onto pregnant women, I wrote *Stress Solutions for Pregnant Moms* to empower women with the tools necessary to identify the warning signs and potential dangers and learn how to deal with them.

This book offers a double benefit: you can reduce the wear and tear on your body during your pregnancy *and* boost your baby's potential for well-being by managing your stress during this critical time. In essence, both you and your baby can benefit from what you'll learn here. Even if you consider yourself to be healthy and under little or no stress, I urge you to review this material and the tools and suggestions I offer here. Why? Simply because many of us aren't good judges of when we are under too much pressure and need to do something to return to a state of balance. When you take the self-assessments in Part Two, you may, in fact, be surprised to see where you fall on the stress continuum. In addition, all of us have days that are more stressful than others and you can use the techniques I share here whenever you need them.

A Three-Part Approach to Prenatal Stress

My approach to addressing the issue of prenatal stress is threefold:

1. *Educate yourself about the problem.*
2. *Learn how to measure your own stress levels.*
3. *Start using a simple new formula and point system to keep your stress levels under control while pregnant.*

I will not be covering typical pregnancy topics such as morning sickness or the "I can't wait until this is over" stage. Many wonderful books along with excellent websites already exist to direct pregnant women through the day-to-day changes in their body and hormones.[1] Instead, my goals in creating this book are to bring together important, cutting-edge information about prenatal stress that every pregnant woman should know and to introduce an easy-to-apply point system, similar to some well-known diet plans, that can be used every day to maintain an optimal prenatal environment in which your baby's development can thrive.

Part One begins with an explanation of the recently discovered connections between chronically high levels of prenatal stress and childhood developmental and behavioral issues. You'll also learn how stress can be amplified for the expecting mom because of the internal changes in her body.

In today's world, where we've come to accept high levels of pressure and nervous tension as "normal," recognizing the degree to which we are stressed is definitely a challenge. Part Two responds to that challenge by detailing how the new formula and daily point system I have developed works. The system calculates how much relaxation and stress reduction you need each day to get back into balance and protect your baby.

As you'll learn in the Stress Solutions Resource Guide in Part Three, there are abundant resources to reduce stress in a measurable way. The resource guide offers many different types of effective, affordable, and readily available solutions to help you return to an optimum state of balance that is beneficial to both you and your child. Many of the tools in that section are things you can start using immediately just by sitting down in your own living room with the guide in hand.

Why Haven't We Heard about This Before?

If prenatal stress is so important, why haven't we heard about this issue before? There are several answers to that question. First of all, the research on prenatal stress is coming out of a new field of study known as fetal origins and maternal-fetal medicine. A growing cadre of professionals is exploring how the environmental conditions during our first nine months in the womb affect the development of our brain and organs. The potential danger of too much prenatal stress has emerged as a significant factor in many published studies. Because this area of research is essentially new, many medical professionals may not be fully aware of the information that is coming to light. It takes time for information on new research to reach the street.

Second, the explanation of how prenatal stress affects the baby is complex. Rather than a simple cause-and-effect situation in which one factor leads to one outcome, several factors come together in complex ways to shape the baby's development in the womb. The complex interactions among the factors predispose a child toward displaying certain behaviors, such as attention deficit disorder or autism. We are actually talking about *risk factors* here, not simple cause-and-effect relationships. One of those risk factors is prenatal stress. On a more hopeful note, because we are talking about risk factors and complex interactions among factors, just having a stressful pregnancy does *not* necessarily mean that your baby will have problems. Other factors could enter the equation to diminish the potentially negative effects of too much stress.

Another reason that information on prenatal stress has not been widely publicized and is just starting to surface in the mainstream media is that the most responsible scientific path is to be sure of results before making general statements. That means, first and foremost, that many different researchers need to come up with the same or similar results and conclusions before scientists are satisfied that a real connection exists. You will see when you review the research later in this book that a large number of studies have now confirmed the connection between excessive prenatal stress and a number of childhood problems.

Finally, you may not have heard more about prenatal anxiety as a factor in your baby's health because of what may be termed an abundance of caution. Some feel that until the medical community can fully agree on a suitable treatment—whether it is a cure, a pill, or a procedure—the research should not be widely publicized. In short, scientists like to be sure that they have medical answers to a problem before rocking the boat.[2]

You can see that it will take many years to gather the kind of information that most scientists require in order to be absolutely certain about all the issues and outcomes related to prenatal stress. However, the magnitude of the problem is potentially astronomical, affecting many millions of current and future women and children. I believe that we should not wait that long to educate women about potential concerns. We can begin now. As with cancer and heart disease, we can take measures to better manage and respond to prenatal stress while we continue to learn more about it. If we can do anything at all to help prepare children to be better equipped to enter society, I believe we are obligated to do it.

The best solutions are often not developed until large numbers of people become aware that a problem exists. As a society, we tend to put our creative minds together to develop solutions once the problem comes to our attention. What better way to galvanize our forces to meet the challenge than to share the research and the possible solutions?

It is my mission in this book to take up the challenge that the research on prenatal stress presents. We should not underestimate the power and determination of expecting mothers to do what is best for their babies. We actually do know quite a bit right now about relaxation techniques that are effective, and we will surely be developing more as people become aware of the need to do so.

Staying a Step Ahead

Early in my career, I participated in the development of the Head Start Program with the Parent Child Development Center. That program was designed to improve a child's potential for academic success through early enrichment. So I have always believed that the best way to deal with most problems is prevention. By putting forth a little effort now to prevent something from happening, we can potentially reduce the number and severity of problems later.

The old adage that *an ounce of prevention equals a pound of cure* is particularly appropriate for the special case of prenatal stress. Of the many factors that have been identified as increasing the risk for childhood problems, some are more difficult to eliminate than others. Conditions of poverty and abuse are harder to tackle, for instance, while risk factors such as smoking can be more easily reduced. Fortunately, the effect of stress on both mother and child is one area where we can make a big impact and where prevention can really make a difference.

I am passionate about sharing this information because I want you to stay as healthy as possible during this beautiful time in your life and, in so doing, boost your baby's potential too. Most of all, I want to help future generations of children be emotionally intelligent, creative, and free from crippling anxiety as they move into their new world.

2

Today's Pregnant Mom Has More to Manage

That the birds of worry and care fly over your head,
this you cannot change; but that they build nests
in your hair, this you can prevent.
—CHINESE PROVERB

A FRIEND WHO was about to become a grandmother for the first time told me of her fears about her daughter's pregnancy. The doctor, she said, was concerned about a premature delivery. My friend confided to me that she was worried that this had something to do with her daughter being a Type A personality and continuing to work long hours at her job. "Could someone under that much pressure," she asked, "expect to have a normal baby?"

My friend wasn't worried about whether her daughter's child would have ten fingers and toes, two eyes and ears, and a nose. She wondered about the baby's disposition, ability to rest, and overall health and well-being. Intuitively, my friend understood what research is now confirming: too much stress during pregnancy, if not properly managed, can affect the baby's development in a number of ways. Stress, for example, is now recognized as a primary factor in preterm birth as well as a number of other childhood problems.[1]

It would seem my friend had reasons to be concerned about her grandchild possibly being born premature. Or did she? Let's explore the terrain and you can decide for yourself.

The notion that modern generations are busier and handle more tasks at the same time than past generations is not only supported by research but is common sense. While we may not need to plow the fields and do the wash by hand, we are juggling more variables, processing more information, and facing increasing psychological demands as our society becomes more technologically advanced. In our fast-paced lives, things change around us rapidly. Change itself is a significant cause of stress because when something in our environment changes, we are compelled to change our behavior. And changing our behavior can be an emotional event often accompanied by fear, anxiety, and even anger.

Our Dangerous Misperception of Stress

We know from years of scientific research that stress can cause or contribute to many physical symptoms or ailments, such as headaches, upset stomachs, muscular tension, decreased sex drive, teeth grinding, tightness in the chest, feeling dizzy, change in menstrual cycle, and erectile dysfunction. Emotional symptoms include lack of interest in doing things you used to enjoy, reduced motivation to complete the things on your to-do list, feeling nervous or anxious, feeling depressed or sad, and feeling as though you could cry for little reason.

To examine levels of stress in the United States and understand its impact, the American Psychological Association (APA) commissioned a nationwide survey in June 2008. The survey gathered information on how the public understands and perceives stress and what people feel are the leading causes of it. The survey also examined common behaviors people use to manage stress. The results of the APA survey call attention to the serious physical and emotional problems associated with stress as well as some other surprising findings.

Well over three-fourths of the survey respondents reported that stress increased their possibility of becoming sick. Over 50 percent of those responding to the survey said that their worries caused them to have trouble falling asleep. Nearly one-half of the APA survey respondents reported that economic and financial woes made their depression worse, aggravated their existing heart disease, and increased their blood pressure. Some 20 to 30 percent of respondents felt that stress led to an increased risk of developing cancer, increased eating of junk food and eating too much, and a reduced ability to make decisions and get things done.

The APA survey also found that stress is rising dramatically in our society and that women are affected more by rising stress than men. Fifty percent of the men and women responding to the survey reported that their sense of distress increased over the past year, and more of the survey respondents reported an increase in physical and emotional symptoms due to stress than the year before. Approximately 30 percent of the people surveyed by the APA rated their stress levels as extreme. Complaints of fatigue and of lying awake at night had increased from the year before (52 percent compared to 48 percent in 2007) and feelings of irritability were up 10 percent from the year before (65 percent compared to 55 percent).

One of the most intriguing findings of the 2008 study

by the American Psychological Association is that despite the fact that we as a society are confronted with more stress today, we have a surprisingly poor perception of how well we are handling that stress. The people who responded to the study reported many physical and emotional symptoms due to stress, including negative effects on their relationships, work productivity, and personal lives. Yet at the same time, the vast majority (81 percent) believed that they are managing their stress very well or somewhat well.

Those two statements are contradictory. On the one hand, people say they are experiencing the increased physical and mental health costs of stress. On the other hand, they say they are actually handling the stress in their lives quite well. This misperception of how well we are really handling stress is an important red flag. It was one of the reasons I designed the easy-to-use system for monitoring stress that you'll learn about in Part Two.

In short, these facts and figures as well as my own experience working with people from all walks of life show that too many of us—including expecting moms—believe that we are handling our busy lives just fine when, in reality, we are not. While we may have come to accept that we live in a frenetic, hassled society, that doesn't make its effects on us any less serious. It only makes our need to address them more important.

How Well Do You Know Yourself?

Let's check back with my friend's daughter and her new baby. As it turns out, my friend's grandbaby seems to be okay after all. She was born close to her expected due date. She does not cry that often and is easily calmed. She loves being held, and picking her up calms her down right away. At four months old, she is sleeping through most of the night.

My friend was a bit sheepish when she acknowledged to me that the baby was fine. She wasn't wrong to be concerned, though. She understands that her daughter was pregnant in a society that is under more stress than when she had been pregnant. It just turned out that her daughter, unbeknownst to her, had actually talked with her OB/GYN about the dangers of prenatal stress. My friend's daughter (I'll call her Madeline) had, in fact, taken special steps to spend a little time each day in the evening unraveling and reducing her stress from the day's activities.

Madeline is definitely an achiever and her mom accurately described her as a Type A personality. Madeline always has many plans to accomplish and goals to meet. She earned a master's degree in anatomy and then went to medical school and became a physician. Each day is full for Madeline and she definitely likes to finish her work list before the end of her day. When Madeline got pregnant, however, she *heard* her doctor's warning not to let her stress build up too much. She did some reading of the new research herself and started examining her life and the events in it to see what she needed to do to reduce extra pressures in her daily life.

One of the things Madeline did when she became pregnant was to examine lists of physical and mental symptoms of stress like the one below. This was the first exercise she did to become more aware of her reactions to the day's events. These aren't the only symptoms of a stressful lifestyle, but hopefully you will find this exercise as helpful as Madeline did. It may help you recognize when your tension is mounting.

Check out these physical and mental symptoms of stress. Do you find yourself . . .

__ Holding your breath under tension

__ Now and then taking a sudden deep sigh

__ Having a racing heart or sweaty palms

__ Clenching your hands or constantly wringing them

__ Being very fidgety or irritable

__ Rapidly shaking your foot or leg while sitting

__ Eating when nervous

__ Feeling wound up like a clock inside

__ Jumping at loud or unexpected noises

__ Having trouble falling asleep

Considering that many people have a misperception of how well they are handling the rising stress in their lives, how well do you know yourself? Did you find yourself checking as many as two or more of the above symptoms? If so, was that a surprise to you?

Madeline was convinced by this checklist to take a careful look at her lifestyle while she was pregnant, and her story shows that working relaxation activities into your schedule can really help. If you checked several of the above symptoms, this is a good time to do something about it. In fact, a major point of this book is that it is important to *stop and take the time to do something to reduce your stress.* If you really do not like to be interrupted in what you are doing, you can skip the exercise below. However, taking a break for even a couple of minutes can usually make you feel better. I've placed a little relaxation break coming up to help you set in motion the act of developing healthy habits of stress reduction.

The key to building any new habit, even taking frequent relaxation breaks, is to repeat the new behavior frequently so that it can become an established pattern or link in your nervous system. Developing a habit basically means that a behavior becomes more or less automatic for you. Various experts offering advice on how long it takes to build a habit agree that it takes frequent repetition for 14 to 21 days. That means you have to be very aware of and conscious of repeating the same behavior each day multiple times. Any person who has made a New Year's resolution to lose weight or start an exercise regimen knows that if you miss even a few days in the beginning of trying to start a new habit, you are probably not going to succeed. The old expression "just wait till next year" may come from that. There is no time like the present to start building a new habit of working with stress solutions. So throughout this book I will remind you to take a break with the following message:

This is a good time to take a relaxation break.

When you see that message, try turning to the Stress Solutions Resource Guide in Part Three and picking out a relaxation technique that you know or something new. As you try the various breathing or music techniques or the simple meditation breaks, you will discover ones that work well for you. You may already have some favorites that you know work well for you. There is nothing magical about the techniques in the resource guide; the benefit is in choosing to take a break. These techniques are based on activities that are known to reduce stress. Your relaxation break only needs to last a few minutes, time enough to take a few breaths and get quiet in your mind.

For this relaxation break, I recommend that you try the Pursed-Lip Breathing Exercise on the facing page. It is a good one to start with and will help to reduce the day's tension that might be building up in your nervous system (see Breathing Resources in Part Three for a complete description). If you don't like this technique, choose another one.

Responsibilities versus Relaxation: the Mental Conflict

My friend, Madeline's mother, is surely not alone in worrying about how much stress her daughter is under and how it could affect her pregnancy. Many grandmothers-to-be recognize that today's generation is busier and is facing responsibilities and psychological demands many times greater than their own generation did. Your spouse or partner, friends, and family may also have concerns about the amount of pressure in your life.

Fortunately, Madeline found a way to reach a good balance between her work responsibilities and personal needs, and she consciously made an effort to reduce her stress daily while pregnant. Unfortunately, some women never find that balance and that can cause major conflict, as you will see in the next example of Stacy.

Like Madeline, Stacy is busy and committed to her career. In contrast to Madeline, Stacy is the kind of person who

Pursed-Lip Breathing Exercise

Step 1: Sit comfortably so that you are able to breathe easily. Usually the most comfortable position for this is lying flat on a pad on the floor or on your bed. Place a pillow or a rolled-up towel under your knees and neck to protect your lower back. (If you are doing a few minutes of breathing and then returning to your reading, set your things down while you take this break.)

Step 2: Close your eyes and become quiet. Breathe normally until you feel relaxed and ready to start.

Step 3: Begin to breathe in through your nose, then puff out your cheeks and slowly blow out your breath through lips that are slightly pressed together. You can accentuate this process by blowing out your air more slowly and for a longer amount of time until your lungs are mostly empty. As you blow out the air, tighten your tummy, as this actually helps make room in your lungs so that you get a nice, deep inhalation for your next breath.

If you are still feeling tense, continue for a few more minutes. Try to stop thinking and just focus on your breath.

does not have a good sense of how stressed she is, and she did not do much to change her busy schedule while she was pregnant. Her attitudes about work and career kept her feeling overwhelmed and responsible on the one hand and conflicted on the other hand because she felt it was important not to overdo while she was pregnant. That is a mental tug-a-war that many career-focused women who find themselves pregnant have to resolve. And it is a hard contest to win without making some basic but doable adjustments.

Stacy is a good example of how we can get worn down by our attempts to live up to all of our responsibilities to family, work or education, and friends and still enjoy a social life. Like so many of today's bright young women, she wants to balance her personal life and her career. Her story, however, indicates that she may not be managing as well as she thinks.

As a lawyer, Stacy has always prided herself on being logical rather than emotional. She uses her cell phone and computer to manage her exercise routine, keep up with her business responsibilities, and watch her diet to manage her weight. She routinely loads up her daily to-do list and has always managed to get most of it done. When Stacy became pregnant, she was excited and intended to revise her daily task list. No more staying at the office until her husband called to find out when she would be getting home. She also planned to start the prenatal yoga exercise class that her OB/GYN recommended.

Adding more to her daily to-do list, though, stretched her even more each day. Thank goodness, Stacy thought, for the modern electronic world at our fingertips. Stacy's plan was to use her cell phone to stay in touch with the office even when she went to yoga class. She set her email on her phone to notify her of important "can't wait" messages. She completely missed the concerned looks that the prenatal yoga teacher gave her whenever her phone would ring and she would excuse herself to go outside the classroom to take the call. Despite her best intentions to relax, Stacy cut her relaxation exercises short to attend to business. Even more problematic was that Stacy could not bring herself to take mental breaks from thinking about what she needed to do next and about business details and issues.

Stacy did not feel particularly bad at any point during her pregnancy, though she did often complain of being overtired and not being able to get all her work done. She didn't recognize that constantly working her to-do list kept her stress level up. As a result of keeping up her fast pace, Stacy's stress levels remained high and unreduced for most of her pregnancy.

Unfortunately, Stacy's story didn't turn out as well as Madeline's. Stacy's baby was born three weeks premature. While there may have been other factors contributing to that, there is a proven connection between too much stress in the early months of pregnancy and preterm birth. Preterm birth presents its own risks for childhood problems, including in-fant breathing problems, health problems, and the challenge of catching up developmentally. Stacy's baby was also hard to comfort. He seemed to fight going to sleep.

One of the key differences between Stacy and Madeline is that Stacy missed the daily symptoms of stress that caught Madeline's attention. To be fair, Stacy is the kind of person who does not have as many of the physical warning signs of too much stress as Madeline does. When Stacy's under a lot of stress, she is not startled by sudden loud noises, nor does she tend to shake or move some part of her body when she is sitting.

Instead, Stacy keeps much of her stress bottled up in her head. Her stress is mostly generated by attitudes and beliefs about work and responsibility. These attitudes and beliefs are like the "birds of worry" in the Chinese proverb I quoted at the beginning of this chapter that can "build nests in your hair" if you let them. The thoughts generated by our beliefs are what trigger the release of stress chemicals in our bloodstream and in our brain. Stacy's fixation on her responsibilities interfered with her ability to relax during her pregnancy, and that likely had an impact on both the delivery and disposition of her baby.

What Stacy needed was a different checklist. Perhaps she would have recognized how stressed she was if she had read a list of attitudes and behaviors to watch out for like the one on the next page. By definition, attitudes and behaviors are deeply ingrained. In other words, most of these are learned over years of our experiences. Once learned, they are not easy to change. If, however, you can be convinced to change your behavior while you are pregnant, you are less likely to return to the same behavior after your baby is born.

If you checked three or more of the items on page 23, you are in the group of people who probably have a moderate to high "baseline" (or starting point) of stress. Did you know that about yourself already? If you didn't, you are far from alone. As the APA survey showed, most people do not accurately perceive how much their demanding lifestyle is affecting them.

People with a baseline of moderate to high anxiety tend

Attitudes and Behaviors to Watch Out For

___ Do you resent stopping before you finish something?

___ Before beginning a project, do you obsessively plan?

___ Would you call yourself a perfectionist?

___ Would others call you that?

___ When you make a mistake, do you have trouble forgiving yourself?

___ When the competition gets tough, do you push even harder to avoid losing, regardless of the consequences to yourself?

___ Would you describe yourself as having a Type A personality or being a workaholic?

___ Do you run out of day before you run out of the things on your to-do list?

___ Do you have difficulty getting an insult or perceived wrong out of your mind?

___ Do you hate being wrong and tend to think and worry about it when it happens?

to think that their anxious or taxing state is normal rather than a condition they need to address. A high baseline of stress could be a result of the accumulated effects of worry on our bodies and our constantly trying to beat the clock. Or it could be a result of being born with a predisposition for anxiety and nervousness. Many people are born high-strung. This means that their system lacks the ability to automatically rebalance itself. Such people are likely to say that they "have always been like that."

The harm that originates with the attitudes and behaviors you might have checked on the list above is rarely felt immediately. The effects accumulate gradually. Stress is not like a broken leg that is impossible to ignore. The pain of a broken leg is immediate and obvious. When we "have always been like that," it is harder to notice when things get worse. Pushing past an aggravation without thinking of the building tension as something we need to fix or change, ignoring how we feel, and going on to the next problem can perpetuate the cycle.

Why Managing Stress during Pregnancy Is Important

Many of us are like Stacy. If you see yourself in her story, know that I wrote this book and developed the stress solutions system with you in mind. Madeline obviously did not need as much convincing of the importance of keeping track of her accumulating stress as Stacy did.

Since Stacy is a young, healthy, and active woman, she is probably able to deal fairly well with stress. Yet it is not Stacy who is the one immediately affected by her busy schedule and busy mind. It is her baby. Stress negatively affects adults, too, but the developing baby is more sensitive to stress than the mother. It can take years for the damages due to stress to show up in an adult, but stress can harm a developing baby in a few months.

That's why the message of this book is that it's important to manage your stress while pregnant to protect your baby during this critical period of development. As you will learn in upcoming chapters, making simple changes in your life-style to reduce your daily stress can have long-lasting benefits to both you and your child.

3

What Busy Schedules and Busy Minds Do to Us

BUSY SCHEDULES ARE a common affliction today. That is a fact of life in the 21st century. Along with a full docket often comes a busy mind, a sure sign of impending stress. Another fact of life, though we may not realize it, is that the busier we become, the more we pay the price in our health and well-being. The next few pages are designed to explain how stress works to trigger physical changes in your body—in other words, how busy schedules lead to busy minds and how busy minds lead to changes in your brain and body over time.

Not long ago, physicians considered diseases that are sensitive to or related to stress to be, at least in part, psycho-somatic—that is, "mostly in our heads." Traditional medicine in the early to mid-1900s did not understand the actual mechanism by which a thought or feeling could cause a heart attack or some other stress-related illness. A feeling or a thought is not physical, after all. That put stress-related illness in a strange position. Since there was no known cause, except for having stress or crazy thoughts, there was less interest in finding solutions to stress-related conditions.

Medicine has come a long way and now better understands that thoughts and emotions, especially stressful ones, actually cause hormones to be released. The hormones enter the bloodstream and communicate the "dis-ease" to specific parts of the body. Ultimately, if the hormones are released frequently and stay in the system too long, they cause known physical problems or diseases, such as insomnia, heart palpitations, or digestive problems. In sum, we now understand that *psycho* (in the mind) – *somatic* (reaction in the body from our thoughts and feelings) is a real phenomenon that can affect our health and longevity.

When the connection was first made between stress and illness, the medical community did not realize the extent of the effects of stress. Today we know that the effects are far-reaching. If we could be busy and think and worry and fume and talk and create all the time with *no* problem, we would not even be discussing this. Unfortunately, that is not the case. My goal in this book is to convince you that taking breaks in activities that produce stress-related hormones is essential if you are going to avoid the long-term effects of too much stress. And taking short breaks is *critical while you are pregnant*.

Busy Schedules Usually Result in Busy Minds

It is theoretically possible to have a busy schedule and not have a busy mind. Someone could move through a busy routine without having to do much thinking or having concerns.

It's more likely, however, that if you have a busy schedule, you are mentally active—thinking, planning, deciding, choosing, and doing a host of other things necessary to stay on schedule. If you look at your watch often, you likely have a busy schedule. If you use electronic aides to keep track of your appointments or your to-do list, you most likely fall into the "busy schedule and busy mind" category. Sometimes a busy schedule can be better described as a group of daily hassles—errands or situations that need your attention.

Some of you might be saying, "Okay, so what? Those things are just a part of life." Well, the problem is that all of the above mental activities automatically cause your brain and body to produce cortisol and other stress-related hormones, such as adrenaline, to varying degrees. It is not really possible to be actively thinking, planning, deciding, choosing, or judging *without* raising the cortisol levels in your system. This is particularly true if you feel the pressure of time or feel that you have to struggle to do something you consider challenging or hard to do. Even doing things like adding up grocery costs in your head as you shop can raise your cortisol to some extent, even though you probably would not be aware of being particularly stressed.

To be clear, you don't become stressed by doing something simple like brushing your teeth. Many of your daily activities are routine and you can easily handle more than one task at once (such as folding the laundry or cooking while watching TV or talking on the phone) with no rise in your stress levels. But running out of time to finish a report or rushing to meet a deadline for your loan application is a different thing. Just thinking about a talk you have to give at the garden club can measurably increase your cortisol levels.

The Danger of a Busy Mind
without a Busy Schedule

What if you don't have a busy schedule? You can still have a busy mind that never stops. That, too, raises your cortisol levels. Perhaps you don't have to face the pressures of a demanding job, do not have a long daily to-do list, and do not face a lot of serious problems or hassles. Yet if you naturally tend to hold on to things and mull them over long after the event has passed, you may still be creating a busy mind without the busy schedule.

The mind is an amazing thing. When we review things that have already taken place, cortisol increases. When thinking about things that might happen but have not happened, cortisol also increases. Thus, your body can experience the effects of increased stress hormones with or without a real event ever happening. The implication of all this is that, to a large extent, the negative consequences of stress are directly due to a busy mind.

Certain conditions or situations are more likely to cause chronic or long-lasting busy minds. These include situations where you are angry about something that happened in the past that was out of your control, are afraid that something might happen, or are concerned about the health or safety of a loved one. Two of the worst situations for chronically raising cortisol levels occur when you perceive a serious problem in your primary relationship or you have major financial concerns.

Chronic means that the same problems occur and reoccur regularly. If you are almost always thinking and worrying over a problem or you continue to dwell on the events of the day even after they are over, that is a chronic issue and your high cortisol levels will rarely come down to the level of being relaxed. Cortisol levels do not drop until your mind calms and becomes quiet or still. So the longer you remain mentally active, even if you are lying in bed or sitting in an easy chair, the longer your levels of cortisol will remain high.

The bottom line is that, in a sense, all roads lead to cortisol in that most kinds of mental activity (busy minds) cause an increase in our body's level of cortisol and stress-related hormones. There's nothing wrong with that—our bodies are built to produce cortisol when needed and then move back into balance once the demand is over. It's just important to recognize if that rebalance is not happening automatically so you can take steps to get your body back into balance.

Cortisol: Friend or Foe?

How does cortisol work and why is it something we need to pay attention to? Cortisol, often called "the stress hormone," is a vital hormone with a key role to play. We need it and it is our friend in some situations, but in other circumstances it becomes our foe. Here's how it works.

As our daily demands increase, our body responds by producing and releasing this stress hormone, among other hormones. The release of cortisol happens by way of unseen messages between the brain and the adrenal glands.[1] As cortisol is released, it increases the flow of glucose into the bloodstream. Glucose is converted into norepinephrine and glutamate. Norepinephrine is an important neurotransmitter that helps us think, remember, and be creative. Glutamate is fuel for our cells; it provides the energy necessary to do mental work as well as respond to perceived dangers or challenges.

Table 1 summarizes the ways that cortisol can be our friend in acute or short-term stressful situations or our foe in prolonged or chronic conditions. In its role as our friend, cortisol provides the extra energy and food (from the glucose) in our blood to cope with everyday challenges. It is there to assist us in every difficult task—from activities like thinking hard or worrying over a problem to working on a crossword puzzle or remembering the amount of a check we wrote yesterday. Cortisol is also present when we engage in extreme physical activity or exercise, give a presentation or performance, have a fight with our boss or spouse or an argument with our child, rush so we are not late for a meeting, or respond to a fall or injury. If we are facing a life-and-death issue, cortisol can also be our protector. It provides us with the energy we need to protect ourselves. It maintains balance in the body when we are under duress for short periods of time.

However, when we experience a number of difficult situations—like a day of grueling meetings at work followed by getting upset over being stuck in an evening traffic jam, further compounded by worrying over family problems once we get home—cortisol may stop being our friend and become our foe. That is particularly true if we continue to think about and be bothered by what happened during the day long after the events are over. The person who is always thinking and worrying may be more susceptible to the negative effects of too much cortisol.

TABLE 1. Cortisol: Friend and Foe

Cortisol is your FRIEND in acute or short-term situations:	*Cortisol is your FOE in prolonged or chronic situations:*
Provides a burst of energy in an unsafe situation	Can make it difficult to sleep or relax
Provides energy during a situation by releasing glucose or sugar into the blood	Causes insulin resistance and the inability to release stored energy and lose weight
Heightens memory	Inhibits or blocks access to memory and damages main memory storage site
Boosts immune system	Depletes immune system

Just as there are two sides to cortisol's effects on us—friend and foe—there are two phases to its activity. It is nature's intention that every cortisol release be followed by a sufficient phase of recovery. In other words, your nervous system was designed to stay in balance by switching to the fight-or-flight mode when you have something difficult or demanding to do, and then once the challenge is over, disengaging that system while turning on the relaxation system to reduce the built-up cortisol. When life was less intense and busy, that is how our nervous systems worked. In today's world, however, many people do not feel that they have the time to take breaks and relax.

What Chronically High
Levels of Cortisol Do to Us

When cortisol and other stress hormones are active or when your nervous system is in fight-or-flight mode, many normal body functions are put on hold. For instance, growth and reproductive activities are inhibited. There is reduced blood flow to the skin and the immune system is less active. Thyroid function is decreased. Blood sugar is increased. Those are short-term adjustments that your body should perform normally; and your body fully expects to reverse those adjustments the minute a crisis or challenge is over.

What happens if you do not take that relaxation break and your busy schedule or busy mind just keeps on working? If the cortisol levels continue to be high for too long, physical problems can begin to develop. Having a busy mind all the time can bring on problems like indigestion, trouble falling asleep, being aggravated when you are interrupted while doing something, gaining weight you find difficult to lose, getting startled at an unexpected loud noise, sighing frequently, or even feeling so overwhelmed that you are close to tears. Those are the type of signals you will look at in Part Two to measure your baseline levels of stress and physical reactivity at the time you became pregnant.

As we get older, chronically high hormone levels can eventually affect our memory and attention, lower our immunity, and reduce the ability of our body to use its inflammatory response to heal wounds efficiently. Prolonged levels of high cortisol can reduce bone density and muscle tone and increase blood pressure as well as suppress the ability of the thyroid to work. These increased levels of cortisol also put a higher demand on the pancreas to produce more insulin in order to activate the body's cells to convert sugar to energy and can produce conditions such as metabolic syndrome or the predisposition toward diabetes.[2] Further, chronic stress and its constant sidekick, cortisol, is a significant contributor to many diseases, including coronary artery disease, heart attack, stroke, small vessel disease, some forms of cancer, insulin-dependent diabetes, chronic fatigue syndrome, delayed hypersensitivity reaction, and many forms of gastrointestinal problems.

Even if you do not have such problems right now, that doesn't mean the effects of prolonged stress will not eventually catch up to you as you age if you don't start taking regular relaxation breaks. We all know of people who worked for years in a high-stress job and seemed to be managing fine— until they retired. They were looking forward to finally enjoying life and having time to relax. Then sometime shortly after retiring but before that long-awaited vacation and life of leisure, they have a heart attack or a crippling stroke or develop cancer.

A well-known theory by Hans Selye explains why this sometimes happens.[3] Selye, an early pioneer in researching the biological effects of stress, called his theory the General Adaptation Syndrome and he outlined several states the individual passes through once under pressure. First, we enter the alarm state, where the body appraises the situation and prepares to fight it. The alarm state is followed by the resistance state, which can last for a long time as the individual fights the situation.

Finally, the body enters an exhaustion state as its resources to fight are exhausted. In such a situation, there can be a period of several months during which the body is more susceptible to disease. This happens because the immune-system resources we need to stay safe from any disease or invading organisms have been suppressed and exhausted in the battle and the body has not had time to recover them. If we retire from a stressful job while we are in the exhaustion state and the stress stops abruptly, the body has dropped its guard and is not able to fight.

One of the benefits of youth is the resilience of our systems. When we're young, we can usually manage things that become problems as we age. As we get older, the possibility that our worries and anxieties may actually contribute to an illness or disease is greater, and we can reach the exhaustion state more quickly.

Most adolescents, for example, don't think twice about staying up late to study for exams. They can pull all-nighters without much more than a yawn the next day. The extra effort and loss of sleep is usually forgotten by Saturday night. As we move into our 20s and 30s, a chronic state of nervous tension and worry can leave us more susceptible to sleeping problems and digestion problems. By the time most of us are in our 40s, if we stay up all night, we need several nights of sleep to catch up. If we have trouble catching up on our sleep or we miss a deadline or if a business trip is not going well, it can cause heartburn, tight muscles, a headache, or worse. If we lose the contract we were counting on, we might well fume about it for weeks. If we lose our job over it, we may face even more emotional, mental, and financial stress.

For some of us, by the time we are in our 50s, life's constant pressures have exacerbated the threat of diabetes, heart trouble, and many other physical or emotional problems. The residual damage has built up in our systems and our body has never fully recovered. As we enter our 60s, a lifetime of stress and anxiety can cost us dearly.

The strain and excesses of years build up slowly. Physical changes and health crises take many months, usually years, to unfold. We don't see the effects coming until they are upon us. By not reducing the overload as the stressful events happen, we risk developing troublesome conditions as we age. A great example of this is what happened to President Bill Clinton. His fast-food diet, coupled with the extreme pressures of the affairs of state, surely contributed to his cardiac problems after he left office and his stress level dropped abruptly.

The current research on the effects of stress and anxiety on aging is very convincing.[4] In addition to physical problems, the studies also show that experiencing significant amounts of chronically high cortisol and anxiety over a lifetime actually predicts the loss of brain tissue in the area of the brain (hippocampus) that is responsible for our long-term memory functioning, new learning, and visual-spatial reasoning.[5] Thus excess stress over a lifetime also contributes to what we call aging memory loss.

What Nature Really Intended

Let's contrast the chronic scenarios I've described above with how a normal, well-functioning nervous system works when we learn to balance our work and play well. People who have a system that is properly functioning naturally seem to do a good job of releasing daily stresses, and their anxiety and stress can be very transient—here one minute, gone the next. They are good at letting go of stress-producing thoughts and feelings. They release mild and short-lived aggravations during the day and don't give these issues much thought again.

If your body does not respond like that or you are the kind of person who has a busy schedule, a busy mind, or both, you will benefit greatly by taking heed and doing something about the stresses and cortisol that build up each day. An effective way to avoid a buildup of high levels of hormones in your system is to take frequent short breaks during the day. To be effective, these need to be breaks in thinking.

Remember the two women in the last chapter? Taking quick breaks is what Madeline did and what Stacy, unfortunately, did not do. Madeline did make some changes in her work schedule and to-do list while she was pregnant, but mostly she learned to take frequent breaks where she simply let her mind relax. These breaks were not long—sometimes only 5 or 10 minutes every couple of hours—but they helped her meet her all-important goal of lowering her stress levels and finding a bit more peace of mind.

This is definitely a good time to take a relaxation break.

4

The Alarming Rise
in Childhood Disorders

*Anxiety always cripples intelligence; it blocks the development of . . .
the ability to interact with the unknown and unpredictable.
. . . Its roots are deep, its branches prolific, its fruit
abundant, and its effects devastating.*
—JOSEPH CHILTON PEARCE, *THE MAGICAL CHILD*

ADULTS ARE NOT the only ones experiencing the effects of
stress and anxiety. More and more, our children are suffer-
ing from these conditions as well. In 1977, Joseph Chilton
Pearce identified anxiety and stress in children as a concern in
his book *The Magical Child*. He warned that anxiety among
our children is a growing problem. Even then, Pearce and
others knew how potentially damaging anxiety can be to
children's emotional and cognitive growth and development.
Pearce believes that anxiety and stress interfere with normal
brain functioning and kill our children's potential to become
all they can be.[1]

We are paying the price now for our lack of vision in
not confronting this issue much sooner. Anxiety is a rapidly growing clinical diagnosis among children. Many more
children suffer from a poor ability to cope with stress—a

condition that is almost never treated, as it is not a clinical diagnosis. Stress-related disorders are increasing from generation to generation. One of the big impacts anxiety has is that it limits new learning and the retention of information in children as well as adults. Think about it: if you are mentally busy worrying about one thing, how can you really focus on something else?

Along with stress and anxiety, depression and other mental disorders are also on the rise among children. More children than ever before are being diagnosed with attention deficit disorders and being put on medication.[2] Autism has received more attention recently than it has since the disorder was named in 1943. In a world that is becoming progressively more attentive to emotional and behavioral disorders, we are counting our children among those in need of therapy and treatment in much larger numbers.

Further substantiation of that fact came from a recent continuing education course I attended at an American Psychological Association convention. The course was taught by Dr. Cecil Reynolds, who described a study done at the University of Texas to update the norms for a popular child evaluation measure, the Behavioral Assessment Scales for Children (BASC). Dr. Reynolds is a clinical psychologist from the University of Texas and one of the creators of the BASC.

The University of Texas research team found that approximately the same number of children had school learning problems as in the initial study 10 years earlier. One thing, however, was significantly different and quite surprising to the research team: the number of children with anxiety disorders increased significantly in that same period of time. In addition, more boys than girls are now being diagnosed with anxiety disorders. At the conference, Dr. Reynolds appeared perplexed when he described the huge increase in childhood anxiety over the past decade. Yet this increase is consistent with other reports that at any given time approximately 1 out of every 8 children meets the criteria for at least one anxiety disorder.

It has been proven that children affected by anxiety do more poorly in school, are more likely to miss out on important social events, and are more likely to become involved in substance abuse. Anxiety can often occur at the same time with other problems, such as depression, eating disorders, and attention deficit disorders. Nearly one-half the number of children with anxiety disorders also suffers with depression.

It's hard to ignore the fact that almost 10 percent of our children from preschool to adolescence suffer from childhood anxiety. Since anxiety in children is easy to overlook, few cases are ever diagnosed or treated. These children may struggle through their lives without ever realizing that the feelings they have and the way their bodies and minds react to stressful situations is treatable or could be avoided.

A recent article by Dr. G. J. Emslie published in *The New England Journal of Medicine* reported that anxiety in young children is hard to treat and easily missed.[3] Nevertheless, Dr. Emslie cautions that we must treat childhood anxiety, which is now reaching epidemic proportions. Untreated anxiety in the pediatric population is devastating to society's growth, since anxiety robs new generations of creativity as well as the ability to think clearly and solve problems under pressure. Once the human nervous system learns to respond with anxiety in a stressful situation, it is hard for it to unlearn or reverse that learned response. As children who are burdened by such problems grow up, anxious and depressed, our societies will lose the gifts those children might have otherwise given.

The Subtleties of Childhood Anxiety

What makes the topic of childhood anxiety so difficult to grasp and deal with is that it can take many forms. You may see it as a child's reluctance to attend a party, not wanting to go to school, fear of sleeping in his or her own bed, or worrying about being separated from a parent (separation anxiety). Other indications of childhood anxiety are a child's nervousness about being in a certain situation or about being with someone he or she does not know (social anxiety); excessive worry about a test, a relative, or about something happening at school; having a nervous system that is easily stressed with a nervous tummy; or having trouble falling asleep and staying asleep (generalized anxiety).

Because anxiety can be hard to identify in very young children, it may be missed by well-meaning and attentive parents. A mother who recently visited my office described her five-year-old child on a kindergarten questionnaire as being "confident and outgoing." In further discussion with the mother, I discovered that the child really never gets excited about going to a friend's party and that she often gets a stomachache when she is there. At a recent birthday party of a neighborhood playmate, other mothers expressed concern when they noticed that the little girl had removed herself from the other children and sat quietly alone.

Although her mom does not recognize it, her young daughter has social anxiety—that is, she is very uncomfortable in social or new situations. She may also have some components of separation anxiety. She prefers to be at home or in a situation with which she is familiar. That way she can avoid feeling so anxious.

Why Are Childhood Problems on the Rise?

The facts and issues you've read about here bring us full circle to the question that started me on the journey of writing this book: *Why are children today bearing the burden of so many more emotional problems, such as anxiety and depression, as well as attention problems and other developmental disorders?* The answer, of course, is compound.

One factor is that anxious parents often pass these behaviors on in the way they interact with their children. If parents are stressed and suffer from conditions of anxiety or depression, their children will often adopt some of the same patterns of behavior as they grow up. Children can learn to fear certain situations or things (like dogs or thunder and lightning) just from watching their parents or other siblings. So the fact that parents are more stressed or fearful is very likely affecting their children.

Research has shown that parenting styles also account for some behaviors and emotional problems in children.[4] For example, parenting styles that primarily use fear and punishment to control a child's behavior can lead to behavioral problems and heightened anxiety in the child. Without realizing it, parents can sometimes create or increase their child's anxiety. Here's a case in point. Many parents' first reaction when their toddler gets too close to the street is to holler loudly at them and then lecture them about the dangers of cars and the street and how they can be killed or maimed and so on. Of course it is imperative that our children be kept safe. It is not likely, though, that a toddler will even understand what you tell them.

A better way to get the message across to very young children without using so much fear is to stay right beside them when they are outside and approaching a street. Yells are not necessary if you are there with your hand in theirs. And dire warnings do not really work to stop the unthinking behavior of running toward the ball as it rolls into the street. As children get a bit older they will understand your verbal warnings, come to recognize the dangers, and learn by example.

Another factor contributing to the rise in childhood emotional problems comes from the environment in which children grow up. Sadly, conditions of neglect, abuse, and/or poverty contribute to the development of anxiety and depression. Children can develop anxiety or a host of behavioral problems as a natural result of these situations. They can also suffer a frightening or intense event, such as being bit by a dog or getting burned, that triggers a panic or anxiety reaction anytime they encounter the same or a similar situation.

You may be wondering about whether nicotine and alcohol are also factors contributing to the rise in childhood emotional problems. It's true that smoking or drinking during pregnancy increases the risk of attention deficit disorders as well as the risk of low birth weight and preterm delivery.[5] The many negative effects of smoking and drinking during pregnancy are well known, however, and more women today than ever before are actively avoiding those behaviors while pregnant. Thus, while smoking and drinking are still important concerns, it would be hard to see them as factors that are causing the *rise* in childhood problems.

What about genetics and biology? We do know that people are predisposed to depression if their parents or grandparents have a history of depression. In my practice, I have definitely seen how anxiety can show up from generation to generation. It is also true that panic disorder tends to run in families. Yet science has not yet uncovered a gene or identified a specific mechanism whereby anxiety is inherited. Biological causes of anxiety do exist (for example, medication-induced anxiety or anxiety resulting from exposure to various toxins), but they are less often seen in young children. Some illnesses (such as asthma and a fear of not being able to breathe) and heart conditions (such as arrhythmia and mitral valve prolapse) can also cause increased anxiety.

While the factors I've named here may play a role in the increase in childhood anxiety and related developmental problems, they do not tell the whole story. Evidence strongly points to another important factor: prenatal stress and anxiety. As our society has stepped up the daily stressors in our lives, we could logically say there has been an increase in the stress and anxiety expectant mothers have to cope with, too, which in turn could be contributing to the increased development of anxiety-related disorders in our children.

Starting in chapter 6, I'll be highlighting the most important new discoveries on the impact of prenatal stress and anxiety. You'll learn about the early studies that led the way to investigations into how prenatal stress increases the risk of developmental problems and anxiety in children. I want to repeat that the reason to pay attention to this emerging new research is not to add more stress or an additional list of dos and don'ts into your already busy life. Instead, I urge you to see this as an exciting discovery that will further empower you in your childbearing years and beyond.

In fact, learning how to reduce your stress while pregnant and respond to emotional challenges in a healthy way can benefit you and your child for many years in many ways. It can benefit you in your relationship with your partner and dramatically improve your quality of life. You can even teach some of the simple-to-use techniques I offer here to your children. As our world becomes more technologically, financially, and vocationally challenging, our children will also need to be able to respond effectively to stress as they grow and mature.

It's always good news when we learn ways to help our children grow up to be healthy and strong. We've known for quite a while that many things a woman does while pregnant can affect the child in her womb, and these recent studies only reinforce that notion. Learning more about how mother and child are interconnected during pregnancy—sharing their lives in a supremely intimate way—means that expecting mothers can take an even more active role in boosting their baby's potential.

Hindsight without Regret

The fact that prenatal stress impacts our children is relatively new information. When my mother and yours were pregnant with us, they did not know about this. Nor did I have any understanding of this when I was pregnant with my own children. None of us who were pregnant and delivered babies before knowing the information you will review here could possibly be held accountable.

My own mother experienced constant worry during her

pregnancy. She was a war bride. While she was pregnant with me, my father, a young first lieutenant recruited from Texas A&M, had been shipped out to Europe and he was slated to go into the offensive at Marseille. I wasn't yet born, and my mother didn't know if she would be raising me alone or not. I can only imagine what it must have been like to get married to your high-school sweetheart, become pregnant, and have him ship out to war in another country before your first child is ever born. Watching the news, waiting for the mail (in an era of no cell phones or Internet), all the while hoping for news that my father was alive and not injured, must have been intense.

Although my father made it home safely after the war was over, my mother suffered the same experiences of every pregnant war bride. Her experience was no different than that of so many whose loved ones have served or are now serving in the military.

Looking back, I can see that I had an inordinate amount of anxiety growing up and I could never really figure out where it all came from. I also had serious asthma from the time I was born until my college years, when I finally got it under control. No one else in my family before or after me has ever had asthma, and I always wondered why I was born with it. It never dawned on me that my having asthma and experiencing so much anxiety may have been related to my mother's own anxiety while she was pregnant with me. In fact, I didn't realize until several days after I had read the research on this subject as I was writing this book that I had uncovered a small piece of my own history.

Each new age brings in a wealth of new information. Sometimes the conventional wisdom on an issue can even change from one extreme to another. When my children were infants, the prevailing advice to young mothers about whether to breastfeed or not changed more than once. So if you have had a first child or a second and are just reading this book now and thinking back to your other pregnancies, please don't feel guilty. Instead, learn from the new research. Pass it on to other mothers-to-be and family members and friends who are a part of your support network. And be gentle with yourself as you incorporate what you are learning into the daily pattern of your life.

This is a good time to take a relaxation break.

Please remember not to skip over these reminders! Take a few minutes and pick out a relaxation technique from Part Three and try it out. Practice and repetition is necessary to build new habits.

5

The Body's Amazing Changes during Pregnancy

A great joy is coming.
—Author unknown

In so many ways, pregnancy is a beautiful and miraculous time in our lives, made more so by the body's intricate internal adjustments as it prepares the ideal environment for our child. Those changes as well as the extra demands of preparing for the baby's arrival can add more physical and emotional upheaval to our lives than usual. So before we explore the research on prenatal stress, it's important to take a quick look at the amazing changes that take place in the body during pregnancy—changes that make it a time when it's more important than ever to pay close attention to how our body responds to stress.

The changes in our internal environment while we are pregnant are nature's way of preparing our bodies to carry, nourish, and ultimately give birth to our children. During pregnancy, the heart and kidneys have to work harder because there is a 30 to 50 percent increase in the volume of blood flowing through the body. The heart pumps faster, the kidneys work harder to filter more blood, and urine output increases. In addition, the baby's size and weight put downward pressure on the bladder and increase the frequency of urination. As the output of the heart increases, the body experiences an increase in other physical pressures as the baby gets bigger inside the mother's body. The uterus grows more than ten times its normal size and holds a thousand times more weight than it holds when it is not pregnant.

Oxygen consumption increases by 20 percent to feed the extra volume of blood. Just as the lungs begin to work harder, the volume of space in the mother's body occupied by the baby begins to increase. This interferes with the ability of the lungs to expand since the diaphragm is pushed up by more than an inch and a half. The upward pressure on the diaphragm and the stomach can cause heartburn and gastric distress. The weight of the baby slows down the passage of fecal matter through the mother's colon. Hormonal changes slow down her ability to digest food. As the diaphragm is pushed upward, the breast tissue enlarges and increases downward pressure on the stomach and diaphragm.

In addition to these physical stresses, the cascade of hormones flowing through the body of the expecting mother can cause nausea early on in the pregnancy. The key role of these hormones is to relax the space inside the mother to allow room for the baby to grow. They help create the internal environment that provides the optimum mix of nutrition for the baby's health.

Hormone Changes and Stress

Hormone changes in response to pregnancy are far-reaching, affecting many systems of the body. These changes are much more complex than I will describe, as that level of detail is beyond the scope of this book. For those kinds of details, the most up-to-date and authoritative reference on pregnancy and childbirth is *Your Pregnancy and Childbirth: Month to Month*, written and compiled by the American College of Obstetricians and Gynecologists, now in its fifth edition (available in English and Spanish).[1] What's useful for you to understand here is how some of the basic hormone changes contribute to the physical stress on the expecting mother.

Let's start with the placenta. The placenta is the interface between mother and child. It allows the flow of nutrients into the baby and the flow of toxins out of the baby without mixing the mother's and baby's bloodstreams. The placenta, directly and indirectly, is also a hormone-making machine. It produces estrogen and progesterone on its own and also signals the ovaries to produce more estrogen and progesterone.

The progesterone and estrogen produced by the ovaries and placenta are vital. Progesterone helps make space for the baby within the womb by relaxing the mother's joints. In that way, progesterone can be a contributor to reducing hip joint pain and low back pain as the pregnancy progresses. Progesterone also relaxes smooth muscle (muscle that contracts involuntarily, which is found in areas like the blood vessels, digestive system, esophagus, bladder, and uterus). Because of its action of relaxing the muscles of the esophagus, progesterone also contributes to heartburn and reflux during pregnancy.

Estrogen plays a role in increasing the amount of blood flow to the uterus and stimulating the production of another hormone, called prolactin, to produce breast milk. The busy placenta also stimulates the thyroid to produce more hormones, which can cause an expecting mother to perspire more and her heart to race at times. The interactions between the three organs involved in the body's important HPA axis (the hypothalamus, pituitary, and adrenal glands) are also affected during pregnancy. The HPA is the three-way master hormonal circuit in our bodies. The interactions between its three organs respond to stress, help us rest and sleep, facilitate digestion, and regulate our immune system, our moods and emotions, and our ability to store energy and then access it.

The hypothalamus, about the size of a walnut, sits in the middle of the brain. It is like a conductor, directing many of the other organs of the body to do their jobs. As well as being responsible for regulating our cycles of rest and sleep, the hypothalamus also regulates hunger, thirst, and our body temperature.

The pituitary gland, sometimes called the "master gland" because it controls the other endocrine glands, lies just under the hypothalamus in the brain. Its job is to maintain a stable environment in the body. The pituitary enlarges nearly 135 percent when a woman is pregnant. This alone is testament that the job of maintaining stability in the body of an expecting mother is more than double what it normally is.

The adrenal glands, which sit on top of the kidneys, produce adrenaline, a hormone that is released into the body to help it cope with mental or physical stress. During pregnancy, the placenta stimulates the adrenal glands to release more aldosterone and cortisol, which has the effect of regulating fluids but which often causes fluid retention.

As the pregnancy develops, cortisol levels increase and they get higher still in the last stages of birth and delivery. In fact, cortisol levels increase up to two to three times during pregnancy—an amazing increase. After delivery, mom's cortisol levels fall slowly over several days.[2]

External Pressures

The changes I've been talking about here are all natural, and the body is designed to handle them. What happens inside the body isn't the only change that takes place during pregnancy, though. Consider all the lifestyle changes required during pregnancy while expecting moms also have to deal with personal and household management, choosing a doctor, scheduling and traveling to appointments, working through the details of the delivery, planning for how the household will change, and preparing for the baby's needs and room.

In addition, more women are working outside the home during much of their pregnancy, so they face the additional stressors of keeping up with job duties, thinking about the realities of maternity leave, traveling to work, and so on. In reality, we should call a pregnant woman who is also holding down a job or taking care of a family a Superwoman. And, yes, I know that the prevailing socially acceptable position is that many of these Superwomen do not want to be treated any differently when they are pregnant.

The middle position I'm suggesting here is that it's wise to pay a little extra attention to stress levels during this delicate period of your life. The combination of internal changes and external pressures while pregnant simply means it's more essential than ever to check in with yourself. If you can determine when your stress levels are high, you can take the necessary steps to reduce the potential effects of that stress on yourself and your child.

Our cortisol levels can be measured by a saliva or blood test, but obviously it's not convenient, practical, or even possible to have saliva and blood tests all the time while pregnant to make sure you are staying in a safe margin with stress and cortisol. The notion of having a simple system for checking cortisol levels, as diabetics do for checking their blood sugar levels, would revolutionize how all of us go through our days. Although many people will profit from such a measuring system, pregnant women are the ones who will benefit most.

Without either a saliva test or a blood test, it is hard to tell for sure what your cortisol levels are. Clearly, until someone invents a simple way of checking cortisol levels, we need another way to do it. That's exactly why I designed the stress-reduction formula and point system you'll learn about in Part Two. It's easy to use and incorporate into your daily routine.

From the short summary in this chapter, you can see why your body during your pregnancy is delicate and therefore sensitive to any additional burden of stress. Dealing with the body's physical and emotional changes, balancing the interplay of hormones, and juggling daily responsibilities can make it easier to reach the tipping point of your internal stress meter while you're expecting. At no other time in your life, then, is it as important to watch and gently manage your stress levels. For as you'll find out in the next chapters, how you handle stress while you are pregnant can affect your child for years to come.

This is a good time to take a relaxation break.

6

Landmark Studies on Pregnancy and Stress

Some scientists have suggested that prenatal stress should be viewed alongside smoking and alcohol intake in pregnancy in terms of its potential adverse effects on the fetus.
—Dr. Thomas O'Connor, University of Rochester

Even though concerns about the effects of too much stress during pregnancy go back to at least the 1950s, they were still dismissed as old wives' tales by many. The research just was not convincing enough to cause people to make big changes in their behavior—until now. We now have scientific proof about the impact of high levels of stress during pregnancy. The breakthrough discoveries in this field are so significant that I've devoted this and the next chapter to summarizing these key findings.

As with many valuable medical discoveries, growing evidence from animal studies led the way to human studies on prenatal stress. Of course, the results of animal studies cannot be directly generalized to humans, but such studies play an important role in pointing us to areas where research with humans is needed.

In early studies, observers discovered that baby animals

born to mothers who were experimentally stressed while pregnant displayed unusual behavioral and emotional characteristics as they grew. The primary finding from these early studies was that the offspring exhibited behaviors in social situations that were very different from the behaviors of normal animals.[1] Some examples of unusual behaviors observed in these early experiments included the offspring freezing or being unable to move out of danger when frightened, being afraid to leave their mother's side and explore when in a new and strange environment, and clinging to the mother. The offspring of stressed animal mothers also displayed decreased ability to learn, mildly delayed motor development, and shorter attention spans than normal babies. In addition, they displayed atypical sexual and mating behavior.[2]

On a more positive note, scientists conducting the studies discovered that while chronic stress (constant or recurring) during the animal's pregnancy had damaging effects on the offspring's development, a short or infrequent period of stress did not appear to adversely affect behavior and development. That suggests that animals are resilient enough to handle short periods of stress. I believe humans are as well. This finding, then, implies something very important: *If pregnant women can learn to manage their stress so it does not become long lasting and chronic, it may be possible to prevent or reduce the potential harm to our children from prenatal stress.*

Linking Prenatal Stress to Childhood Behaviors

The findings that emerged from the early animal studies were so strong that researchers naturally wondered whether human babies would show the same negative impact from prenatal stress. Think about it. The atypical animal behaviors of the offspring of stressed mothers that affected their learning, social development, and emotional behavior are similar to certain maladaptive behaviors seen in some young children who are more than normally cautious about leaving their mother's side or refuse to talk to or play with other children or adults. Parents are always concerned when their toddler refuses to talk to or acknowledge other people they meet or when the child clings to them and refuses to explore a new, fun place. Some of these children are also easily frightened, just as the animal offspring of chronically stressed mothers were.

I have met many parents in my practice who are afraid to tell their toddler no when the child asks for a snack before dinner for fear that the child will become upset or throw a tantrum. Once upset, these children often cannot be easily calmed. Some will cry until they exhaust themselves, make themselves sick, or finally fall asleep. In essence, these children deal very poorly with interpersonal situations, with novelty of any kind, with learning, and with any opposition to what they want.

Of course, there may be other explanations for the similarities between the emotionally challenged children and the offspring born to stressed animals than the one I'm going to offer. Some people favor an explanation that portrays the maladaptive emotional behaviors in children as simply examples of differences in human temperament (shyness, fearfulness, irritability) or as individual differences in the ability to deal with emotional situations. Recent research, however, strongly points to another explanation for these tendencies: chronic prenatal stress.

Determining if prenatal stress has the same effects on humans as it does on animals presented some obvious challenges to researchers. For one, it is much harder to gather this type of information with humans because we obviously cannot experimentally shock pregnant mothers to see how that affects their babies. At first, researchers had to rely on naturally occurring situations, such as studying children born during World War II in Europe or children born after a major life event like a natural disaster or events such as 9/11.

Many such studies have been done. One example is a study on Dutch women who were pregnant during the five-day invasion and defeat of the Netherlands by the German army in May 1940. Researchers found that the constant pressures on those mothers were related to a significant increase in the chances that their children would become schizophrenic.[3] Another study looked at the children of women who experienced significant emotional trauma and physical hardship during a natural disaster—an ice storm in Quebec, Canada, that left millions with no power for weeks. When the Canadian children reached five-and-a-half years of age, they were evaluated with an IQ test and a test of language skills. The children of the mothers who reported higher levels of emotional upset during the time they were without power scored lower on intellectual testing (Full Scale IQ and Verbal IQ) and on receptive vocabulary abilities when compared to children of mothers who reported low stress from the same event.[4]

What about pregnant women who experience various upsetting conditions in the normal course of living but who did not experience such a traumatic situation or for as long? Do other kinds of prenatal stressors affect the developing child? Are the effects of prenatal stress uniform at all points or times during the pregnancy or do stresses experienced in the first trimester have different effects than stresses in the second or third trimester? We have some early answers to those questions. However, by no means has the scientific community answered all the relevant questions that need to be addressed.

Many of the early studies that started to address these questions were like the Canadian study; they were natural experiments. Natural experiments are not the best way to study such a complex issue as the effects of prenatal stress and anxiety on a child. For one thing, many other possible explanations can usually be put forth to explain the findings of experiments that take advantage of a natural disaster. On the other hand, setting up a thorough study that can rule out most, if not all, alternative explanations is very expensive and takes a long time to finish. Fortunately, a breakthrough opportunity for just such a definitive study came in the early 1990s with the landmark, long-term research project known as the Children of the 90s project.

A Breakthrough Study on What Causes Childhood Problems

The Children of the 90s study, or more properly the Avon Longitudinal Study of Parents and Children (ALSPAC) is the longest-running and largest medical study in the world.[5] It includes approximately 14,000 children born in the Avon area of England (around Bristol and Bath) between April 1, 1991, and December 31, 1992. Estimates indicate that almost 90 percent of the women who were pregnant in that geographical area and in that time frame participated in the study. To date, the ALSPAC project has produced over 100 publications dealing with pregnancy, parenting, and child development. Only by visiting the ALSPAC website can one get a real sense of the scope of this study. In the first eight months of 2011 alone, more than 40 major journal articles covering topics such as genetic markers of obesity in children and sleep-disordered breathing were published.[6]

Why is the Children of the 90s study so groundbreaking? First, it is a *longitudinal* study. That means the same children are followed and studied for a period of time as they grow up. The children of the Avon study are now in their early 20s. This study was also designed to be an *epidemiological* study. Most key public health studies are epidemiological. An epidemiological study deals with the causes, distribution, and control of disease in populations. An epidemiological study is also designed to include all the factors that might be essential in explaining the question that is being studied. The Children of the 90s research is epidemiological because it includes all the aspects researchers thought might play a role in how children develop, including elements such as the mother's health, the environment, parenting attitudes, the home environment, and other factors. That is one reason why the study is so important—it tracks so many variables.

The Children of the 90s study is also a *prospective* study. Rather than taking a group of children who already have problems and then trying to figure out what went wrong in the past, a prospective study starts by selecting a group of pregnant mothers and recording everything thought to be relevant and important to see what develops. Thus, the researchers working on this study are measuring many factors in order to see what predicts health and behavioral problems as well as successes in children as they mature. Because of the compelling results of the animal studies on prenatal stress, the designers of the ALSPAC project included prenatal stress and anxiety as factors to be studied.

Here's a little background on how this project was born. During the summer of 1985 at a meeting in Moscow, the World Health Organization (WHO) decided to create a prospective, longitudinal study using the survey strategy to examine the current problems in child health and development and to explore ways these problems could be prevented. Out of this decision came a study designed to include several sites, or centers, working simultaneously in different European cities. The overall study was called the European Longitudinal Study of Pregnancy and Childhood (ELSPAC).

One of the research sites selected for this endeavor was Avon, England. The Avon Longitudinal Study of Parents and Children (ALSPAC) has built onto and substantially extended the original European WHO project design. This study is still going today. The original research project was designed to follow the mother, her partner, and the child in the study from conception to 7 years of age in a number of European cities. The Avon Children of the 90s study is now following the children into adulthood because its findings have been and continue to be so valuable. This project is, in fact, the world's largest *cohort study*, a term that means that the study includes all the children born in a certain area in a certain time period. Together, the children form a group that shares those key elements or experiences (therefore the term *cohort*).

The Children of the 90s study is an example of an experiment that is so well designed that the results it is yielding are scientifically convincing and credible. The design of this research is the brainchild of Professor Jean Golding, an epidemiologist. The study has been collecting data to document how the children are being raised, what problems they have growing up, and how those problems might be prevented, among many other issues. In essence, the study is aimed at better understanding how to help children reach their full potentials in education, health, and happiness by learning how physical and social environments interact with our genetic inheritance to shape our health, development, and behavior.

Only one part of the mass of data being collected on the Avon mothers and children is designed to answer questions related to what prenatal and postnatal factors are associated with the development of future childhood problems. Many other important questions are being studied and much valuable information has already been discovered. For instance, an important discovery from this huge endeavor concerns lead poisoning and what blood lead levels adversely affect learning and attention. Over 500 children were included in the lead poisoning part of the Children of the 90s study. Whereas both the American and the British governments have set so-called safe levels of blood lead at less than 10 micrograms per deciliter, data from the Avon study actually indicates that the standards could be lowered even further.

Bone density is another health concern examined in the Children of the 90s project. A recent report indicates that teenage girls who are too thin are putting their bones at risk. Researchers have also collected data about the food that mothers ate during pregnancy and discovered that if the pregnant mom eats oily fish during her pregnancy, her child will be born with better eyesight. The scientific community involved in the Avon study is also looking for relationships between aspects of home and community life and the child's growth and development. For example, biological samples have been stored as a means of identifying pollutants and assessing their influence on the child's development.

Harriet is one of the children taking part in this project. As a 2004 article in *The Times* (London) describing this landmark study put it, Harriet "is one of the most influential children in Britain," helping to "shape the way future generations are brought up."[7] As part of the study, Harriet has grown up with researchers closely observing her home and environment, including what she eats, how much toothpaste she uses, what chemicals she is exposed to, the way she is taught in school, how her parents interact with and parent her, and her social and genetic family history. As the Avon study children grew older, researchers asked questions about education and what the children planned to do when they grew up. Harriet said she wasn't sure whether she wanted to become an actress or a cartoonist.

The mothers who volunteered to participate in this study answered questions about their beliefs and attitudes surrounding their pregnancy by completing long questionnaires that they returned by mail at specified times during their pregnancy. These included questions about the sources and severity of stress and anxiety in their lives. Harriet's mother completed several such questionnaires as part of the study when she was pregnant.

For their article, *The Times* interviewed Harriet and her Avon family. Harriet's mom is a teacher. Harriet said she is enthusiastic about the Children of the 90s project. Most of her friends at her school also take part in the ALSPAC study.

62 | STRESS SOLUTIONS FOR PREGNANT MOMS

Harriet said that she used to dislike giving blood, but now she is used to it and she recognizes how much valuable information she and her classmates are providing to the world. There are a surprisingly low number of study dropouts. People who have moved away from Avon even come back annually in order to complete their long questionnaires.

How to Move through
the Research More Quickly

Before I move into more detail about the Avon research and the important information in the next two chapters, I want to offer an alternative for readers who are not interested in the technical details of each study. As one who has spent her life in an applied field of science (psychology), I feel that it is irresponsible to report conclusions without offering some supporting detail about how the writers arrived at their conclusions. Many readers may feel the same way. Others of you may want to move more quickly into the practical aspects of the book.

To accommodate both types of readers—and reduce your stress—I have moved some of the research study details to the endnotes from this point on. Each note is numbered and will be easy to find. If you prefer to skip the notes for now, the summaries of the research in this chapter and the next two will move quickly for you. Chapter 7 shares more about what childhood problems are associated with high prenatal stress and chapter 8 discusses the dynamics in the womb that communicate what the expecting mother is experiencing to her unborn child. Part Two goes on to talk about what to do with all this information. If you want to move ahead to the sections on how to measure and reduce your stress, you can scan the upcoming chapters or skip ahead to Part Two and Part Three and come back to the details later.

ALSPAC Findings on Prenatal Stress

In 2002, the first papers from the data collected on Avon mothers and their children concerning prenatal stress were published.[8] One of these compared the mothers' reported prenatal anxiety levels to the problems their children were having at 4 years of age. Another published article from the same large data bank evaluated whether or not depression might also be a factor in the findings. Researchers found that antenatal (prenatal) anxiety predicts child behavioral and emotional problems independently of the mom's postnatal depression. Those findings were based on data from approximately 7,500 mothers and babies from Avon.[9]

Mothers completed prenatal questionnaires at two time points during their pregnancy (18 weeks and 32 weeks gestational age). The information the mothers provided at those two points included the Crown-Crisp Index of Phobic Anxiety[10] (reproduced on page 70) as well as other information on their health, smoking, and drinking history and statistics about their pregnancy. Postnatal questionnaires about the mothers' levels of anxiety, stress, and depression were gathered when the child was 8 weeks, 8 months, 21 months, and 33 months old. At each of those data collection points, the mothers completed questionnaires rating their children's attention, conduct problems, and emotional adjustment.[11] As the children reached the age of 4, they went through a thorough hands-on evaluation. For the purposes of the study, the mothers were considered "anxious" if their Crown-Crisp anxiety ratings ranked in the top 15 percent.

Scientists from many different disciplines worked on the Avon project. Dr. Thomas O'Connor, a clinical psychologist and a key member of the ALSPAC study team, participated in writing a number of the studies that came out of the Avon research on prenatal anxiety. He was the lead author on the first study I mentioned above that compared the mother's level of anxiety during her pregnancy to how she rated her child's conduct problems, emotional adjustment issues, and problems with attention at 4 years. This first paper, published in the *British Journal of Psychiatry*, reported that mothers who scored in the top 15 percent of anxiety at 18 weeks or 32 weeks gestational age were two to three times more likely to have a child with significant emotional problems, attention problems or conduct difficulties at age 4.[12]

To get an accurate assessment on the question of what best predicts childhood problems, Dr. O'Connor and his team had to be sure they were looking only at the effects of a mother's anxiety *while* she was pregnant and not the effects that her moods might have had on the child *after* he or she was born. They found that including postnatal depression and anxiety in the analyses, measured at 8, 21, and 33 months after birth, did not change the results or the interpretation that prenatal anxiety is strongly related to several problems in child development. In other words, prenatal anxiety is a significantly better predictor of childhood problems than the mother's depression or anxiety after the child is born.

Earlier in the book you read about what causes stress, the different types of stress, and how the effects of mild versus severe stress differ. To put the findings you're reviewing here in context, Dr. O'Connor and his colleagues were reporting on the Avon mothers who said that they experienced a *severe* form of anxiety, and one that more appropriately should be termed *chronic*, when they were pregnant. The highly anxious Avon mothers could be described as overly mentally active, both in terms of their worrying and their thinking. The Crown-Crisp Index completed by the women measures self-reported fears and phobias, such as being afraid of enclosed spaces, fear of heights, or worrying a great deal when a loved one is late coming home. Those kinds of fears and worries do not usually go away once the baby is born. Nor do they begin just because the woman is pregnant.

The problems these Avon women were reporting would have been persistent problems in their lives for a long time and would have already changed the way their nervous systems dealt with stress. These women likely produced and kept more cortisol in their bloodstream than the mothers who were able let go of thoughts and fears quickly.

It is critical, and perhaps obvious, to say that not everyone who lived in Avon and was pregnant from 1991 to 1992 was exceptionally anxious. To keep this information in a good perspective, the numbers indicate that approximately 65 percent of the 7,500 pregnant Avon women reported that they experienced "no anxiety" at any of the data collection points.[13]

Childhood Problems Related to Prenatal Stress Don't Go Away

Another key finding associated with the Children of the 90s study is that the problems children were born with that were associated with the mother's level of stress during her pregnancy did not go away and did not get better as the children aged. Researchers found that the types of problems these children were reported to have at age 4 were still problems as they approached 7 years of age.[14]

In addition, another look at the mass of data collected in Avon showed a direct relationship between the mother's pre-natal cortisol levels and the child's cortisol levels at age 10. As in the earlier study by Dr. O'Connor, he and his team elimi-nated any influence of the mothers' mental health (depression and anxiety after the child was born) as a contributing factor in explaining the increased cortisol found in the 10-year-old children of mothers with high prenatal cortisol levels.[15]

Clearly, the Avon children whose problems were related to their mothers' high prenatal anxiety levels are not growing out of their issues. As you will see in the coming chapters, many studies are now pointing to the same important con-clusion: *moderate to high levels of persistent prenatal stress can result in lasting damage to a child's emotional response system.* Dr. O'Connor is now in the process of initiating a large fol-low-up project in the United States funded by the National Institutes of Health (NIH). In the coming NIH study, ap-proximately 8,000 families will collect saliva samples from their children at age 14 to examine their cortisol levels and look more closely at the mechanisms by which anxiety and stress in pregnancy can have long-term consequences on the intellectual, emotional, and behavioral development of chil-dren and adolescents.

Table 2 provides a summary of the main findings on pre-natal anxiety from the Avon project. The key findings were reported over several articles.

TABLE 2. Key Findings on Prenatal Anxiety from the Children of the 90s Project

1. There is a strong and likely causal relationship between high levels of prenatal anxiety and a child's conduct problems, emotional adjustment issues, and attention difficulties at age 4.

2. Children of highly anxious moms were two to three times more likely to have problems with attention and behavior than children of moms with low anxiety.

3. The findings for #1 and #2 above were not due to the mom's moods after the birth, her drinking or smoking history, age, education, concerns about housing or the pregnancy, or the child's gestational age at birth.

4. As the children got older, the problems with attention, conduct, and emotional difficulties associated with their mother's high stress levels during pregnancy had not gone away.

5. The mother's high stress levels during pregnancy predicted the child's high cortisol levels at age 10. The higher the mother's prenatal cortisol levels were, the higher the child's cortisol levels were at age 10.

Important Take-Home Conclusions

What can we take away from the Avon project's crucial research? One inference from the studies reported in this chapter is that as a mother's levels of stress and anxiety go down, so should her risk of having a child with behavioral, emotional, or attention problems.

Another important take-home point is that having high

levels of stress and anxiety during pregnancy does *not* mean that your child will definitely have problems. The "increased risk" in this case means that *more children from high-stress pregnancies have problems than do children from low-stress pregnancies*. However, it is important to remember that the large majority of the children in the Avon study did not exhibit clinically meaningful problems.

To repeat: this research is *not* saying that stress will always cause problem behavior and reduced emotional adjustment for children later in life, but it does make it more likely. Professor Vivette Glover, an important member of the ALSPAC study team and a professor of perinatal psychobiology, made that point when she said, "It is important to emphasize that this research shows that antenatal anxiety leads to the risk of hyperactivity increasing from one in 20 to one in 10. Not every anxious mum will have a hyperactive child."[16] In a recent review article, Dr. Glover emphasized that mothers-to-be commonly experience mood swings and worry from time to time and that the results we're reviewing here were found in women with much higher levels of anxiety.

Another point to keep in mind is that even though excessive and unreduced prenatal anxiety and stress has been proven to have negative consequences, not all stress is negative. Some types of stress of limited duration may actually be beneficial. By definition, even receiving exciting news can be considered to be at least a mildly stressful event. That kind of event is a frequent occurrence in the normal living of life. It is no surprise, therefore, that mild stresses of certain types make us stretch and grow. But as of this writing, I am aware of only one popular science writer who has recently stated that prenatal stress might be good or potentially beneficial for the baby's development.[17]

In fact, on closer inspection, the studies that support that statement do not define stress in the same manner as the greater proportion of research reviewed in this book. In other words, what is being measured in the studies reporting that stress can be beneficial is a kind of stress that is mild and of short duration. For instance, Dr. Janet DiPietro published a number of studies using healthy women with low-risk pregnancies, usually measuring their fears about the birth process and body changes. The definition of prenatal stress in several of her studies is mild by comparison to the type of prenatal stress defined in the Avon studies.[18]

Conclusions about the relationships between prenatal stress and behavioral and developmental problems can sometimes be overstated and sometimes understated in reports. When exploring the research on your own, please pay attention to the way research studies define and measure prenatal stress, how they measure the effects on the child, and what conclusions they draw from the findings so that you are not confused about what might, at times, seem to be contradictory findings.

How Do You Score?

Since you've been reading so much about children like Harriet and some of the results of the Children of the 90s study that they are a part of, you might like to see the questionnaire (the Crown-Crisp Index of Phobic Anxiety) that was used to measure anxiety and define high levels of chronic prenatal anxiety. You can take a moment to answer these questions yourself on the next page and add up your score.

Crown-Crisp Index of Phobic Anxiety

	0	1	2
1. Do you have an unreasonable fear of enclosed spaces, such as shops, elevators, etc.?	Never	Sometimes	Often
2. Are you scared of heights?	Not at all	Moderately	Very
3. Do you feel panicky in crowds?	Never	Sometimes	Always
4. Do you find yourself worrying about getting some incurable illness?	Never	Sometimes	Often
5. Do you dislike going out alone?	No		Yes
6. Do you feel uneasy traveling on buses or trains, even if they are not crowded?	Not at all	A little	Definitely
7. Do you feel more relaxed indoors?	Not particularly	Sometimes	Definitely
8. Do you worry unduly when relatives are late coming home?	No		Yes

The Crown-Crisp Index is scored 0, 1, or 2 depending on the answers to each question, with a total possible score of 0 to 16. If your total score is over 8, you are acknowledging a high level of anxiety. You should also know that one does not score high on this index one time and low the next. It is not a set of questions for which your answers will change greatly without a lot of work. The questions are asking about beliefs, fears, and attitudes that you have probably had for a long time, which is why they are considered chronic.

Keep in mind that the Crown-Crisp Index measures only one kind of stress—phobic anxiety and fears. Most of the studies reviewed in the next chapters measure a different kind of stress, such as stress resulting from arguments with your partner, financial burdens, and excessive worrying and thinking (the busy mind I described in chapter 3). So it is possible to score low on the Crown-Crisp Index and still have a lot of stress. When you get to Part Two, you'll find other questionnaires that focus more on lifestyle and daily hassles and that will help you easily keep track of your stress levels.

In the next chapter, we'll explore additional solid research that backs up the findings already reported on the effects of high levels of prenatal stress and anxiety. Remember, the reason I am sharing this research is to empower you. The more you know about the risk factors, the better equipped you'll be to take steps to counteract them with the resources provided in Parts Two and Three. Knowledge is indeed power.

This is a good time to take a relaxation break.

7

Childhood Problems
Related to Prenatal Stress

We may not be able to prepare the future for our children,
but we can at least prepare our children for the future.
—Franklin D. Roosevelt

THE LAST CHAPTER examined a progression of valuable research on prenatal stress, from early studies of stress during pregnancy to the world's largest and longest-running study on the factors that can lead to a variety of childhood problems. What has gradually emerged is a clear relationship between highly stressful conditions during pregnancy and problems that arise for the children of the mothers who experienced that stress.

The findings of the Avon study on prenatal stress that you read about in chapter 6 are not isolated. Countless articles are being published in international journals on this topic and the American Academy of Pediatrics issued a landmark warning on January 1, 2012. In their report entitled "The Lifelong Effects of Early Childhood Adversity and Toxic Stress," they reviewed converging lines of scientific evidence that illustrate how different types of stress can leave a lasting mark on a child's developing brain and long-term health.

The American Academy of Pediatrics' position paper acknowledges that the period of time from conception through early childhood is critical. They include prenatal stress in their definition of toxic stress and say that children exposed to early stressful conditions are more likely to struggle in school, have short tempers, manage stress poorly, and tangle with the law.[1]

In this chapter, we'll explore the major findings about prenatal stress to date. One of the easiest ways to describe them is to group the emerging research by the kinds of childhood problems now seen as related to high, chronic, or persisting levels of prenatal stress. At this point, the list of problems that have been investigated is lengthy, with childhood anxiety disorders and the well-known attention deficit hyperactivity disorder at the top of the list. Table 3 provides a quick reference of these problem areas.

TABLE 3. Childhood Problems Associated with Chronically High Prenatal Stress and Anxiety

Attention deficit hyperactivity disorder (ADD/ADHD)

Childhood anxiety and depression

Autism or a developmental problem on the autistic spectrum

Motor developmental delay, poor coordination

Premature delivery or low birth weight

Learning disabilities

Reduced ability to cope with stress (crying, tantrums, freezing, clinging)

Lower IQ

Lower emotional intelligence (EQ)

Unmanaged prenatal stress increases the risk of having a child with one or more of the problems described in table 3. The evidence that links prenatal stress to childhood problems has been growing for many years. The problems themselves aren't new. What is new is that, until recently, these problems were not associated with the mother's level of stress during her pregnancy.

The research also shows that the higher the level of prenatal stress, the greater the risk of problems in children, as diagrammed in figure 1. Please remember as you read that we are talking about *increased risk only*. We can be grateful for the fact that prenatal stress does not always result in childhood problems. In other words, there are probably gradations of problems that can be represented on a continuum from no issues or only minor issues to the major developmental problems that occur under conditions of chronic and severe stress.

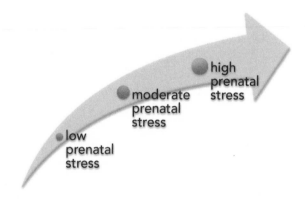

FIGURE 1. The risk of childhood problems increases as the chronicity and severity of prenatal stress increases.

Attention Deficit Hyperactivity Disorder (ADD/ADHD)

In addition to the Avon project, a study from the Department of Psychology at Catholic University of Leuven, Belgium, is one of many that report a relationship between a pregnant mother's high or chronic levels of stress and symptoms of ADD/ADHD, childhood anxiety, and other behavioral problems developing as her child gets older. The Catholic University of Leuven study is a prospective (looking forward) study, which, as I noted earlier, identifies a target group of subjects and follows them over time to see what develops. [2]

The authors of that study found that mothers who reported *more anxiety* during the early part of their pregnancies were more likely to have overly active, hard-to-manage, and anxious children. Those children were also rated as being more likely to overreact to stress and to be diagnosed with ADD/ADHD. The strongest predictor for the development of childhood problems was a higher level of stress and anxiety in the early part of the pregnancy compared to the mother's reported level of stress and anxiety during the last two months of the pregnancy.

Using a careful scientific process to control for other factors, the researchers verified that it was the mother's anxiety levels during pregnancy that best explained the problems they found in the children years later. None of the other factors—such as smoking during pregnancy, the child's birth weight, the mother's educational level, and whether or not the mother was anxious after the birth (postnatal anxiety)—predicted the development of childhood problems as well as prenatal stress and anxiety did. It has long been known that smoking during pregnancy has many deleterious effects, including increasing the risk of a child born to a smoker being diagnosed as having ADD/ADHD. So the finding that prenatal stress predicted problems like ADD/ADHD better than factors like smoking did is especially noteworthy.

Childhood Anxiety and Depression

In addition to higher levels of prenatal stress being associated with the increased probability of ADD/ADHD, high stress during pregnancy is also associated with various forms of childhood anxiety and dysfunctional stress reactions. It has been estimated that anxiety disorders are now affecting anywhere from 6 to 20 percent of children and adolescents. Many studies report and support the relationship between prenatal stress and childhood anxiety.

For example, research shows that children born to moms who were overly stressed while pregnant have a harder time falling asleep than children born to moms who were not anxious and fearful while carrying their children. The children of high-stress pregnancies can also have problems with depression and show exaggerated reactions to stress. They often react with increased stress in novel social situations. Frequent crying or being upset easily, displaying temper tantrums, problems separating from their mothers when it is time to go to school, and extreme fearfulness, shyness, and nervousness in new situations are some of the behaviors that are associated with excessive amounts of anxiety and stress during their mothers' pregnancy.[3]

Earlier, I presented evidence that childhood anxiety is on

the rise for several reasons. Not only is it on the rise, but childhood anxiety is also hard for parents and professionals to recognize and is difficult to treat. Children are not usually able to put words on their feelings of worry or fear. They typically only report physical symptoms such as stomachaches and headaches. Such physical symptoms might mean other things besides anxiety. Avoidance of certain situations and difficulty transitioning from one situation to another are other ways children show their anxiety. These behaviors can also be misinterpreted and the underlying anxiety not recognized or treated.

Autism and Autistic Spectrum Disorders

The causes of autism are becoming better understood. We now know that instead of a single cause of autism, many factors contribute to a range of behaviors and problems that are called autistic spectrum disorder. Several converging lines of evidence suggest that, surprisingly, a mother's chronically high level of stress is one of those factors that increases the risk of her child having autism. While many of the possible factors that contribute to acquiring this disorder may not be easy to identify and control, the good news is that the amount of prenatal stress a woman experiences is both manageable and often preventable.

One excellent review describes over 40 recent articles coming out of prestigious institutions that link prenatal stress to an increased risk of childhood autism.[4] The stressful life events of significance in these studies include household financial stress, death of a loved one, and discord in the mother's primary relationship.

Lower IQ and Learning Problems

Learning problems and reduced IQ are two more issues related to high levels of prenatal stress that are costly to society and hard to fix once they emerge. Several recent studies have been published suggesting that high levels of prenatal stress can decrease a child's IQ by as much as 8 to 10 points.[5]

A loss of 8 points in IQ is potentially much bigger than it might appear. Here's why. An IQ of 100 is at the 50th percentile, meaning that if 100 children were randomly selected, the child in the middle of the group would have a score of 100. If that child lost 8 points, that would bring his score to 92, falling to the 30th percentile, or to the bottom of the Average range. He would move from 50th in the group of 100 to 30th in the same group, or a loss of 20 percentage points.

An even larger potential loss can be seen for children who start with a lower general intelligence, say an IQ of 75 (which is in the 70 to 79 range, called Borderline). A loss of 8 points for these children would make their score 67. Any score below 70 is in the range called Exceptionally Low or Mentally Retarded. At the other extreme, 8 points might make the difference between an adolescent who gets a scholarship for college versus one who does not. So you can see that an 8-point drop in IQ could be significant and could result in a child dropping from an Average to a Below Average level of intellectual functioning.

While a high IQ is certainly not the only determinant of a child's future success, it has relevance. We all want our children to be bright, happy, and successful, and we do whatever we can to help make that happen. It only makes sense, then, to watch your stress levels carefully while pregnant.

Emotional Intelligence at Risk

Emotional intelligence is a relatively new concept that may not be as well known as other childhood issues like ADD/ADHD and autism. Emotional intelligence, or EQ, is a term made famous by Daniel Goleman in his book *Emotional Intelligence: Why It Can Matter More Than IQ*, published in 1995. EQ refers to our ability to handle our emotions and to successfully relate to others in our world. Goleman makes a compelling case for EQ being a bigger determining factor for success in one's job or career, leadership abilities, and coping with adversity than IQ or any other social factor.

You've seen many times now in this book reports of studies showing that behaviors such as being afraid to explore new or strange environments, coping poorly with stressful situations, and avoiding situations that are new or difficult are associated with a mother's chronically high levels of prenatal stress. Those are all behaviors that make up our emotional intelligence. When all the pieces have been counted, it could turn out that emotional intelligence is one of the principle abilities our children lose when prenatal stress is not properly managed.

Reduced Birth Weight, Preterm Birth, and Infant Illness

The list of problems associated with excessive prenatal stress includes a number of problems that can negatively affect the child's physical health, including reduced birth weight, preterm birth, and childhood asthma, to name three of the biggest ones. Reduced birth weight is, of course, closely related to preterm birth. Preterm babies have a higher risk of pulmonary disease, developmental delays, learning disorders, and even infant mortality. Preterm birth is of major concern today and many OB/GYNs are trying to find solutions.

Dr. Calvin Hobel, for example, has spent a lot of his career documenting the effects of stress on pregnancy and developing ways to help pregnant women to relax. He is a perinatologist, a professor of obstetrics/gynecology and pediatrics at the University of California in Los Angeles, and the director of Maternal-Fetal Medicine at well-known Cedars-Sinai Medical Center in Los Angeles. Dr. Hobel has served on many national committees, particularly in the areas of his primary research interests, preterm birth prevention and maternal stress, including the Surgeon General's Committee on Preterm Birth Prevention. Dr. Hobel and the other physicians involved in research to reduce the number of women affected by preterm delivery have discovered that anxiety and excess stress in the first trimester may be setting the clock for early labor. The reason for this is that when a pregnant woman gets anxious, her nervous system releases epinephrine and norepinephrine, which constrict blood vessels and reduce oxygen to the uterus.

Another major factor in the dynamic of prenatal stress and preterm delivery is the placenta's overproduction of corticotrophin-releasing hormone (CRH) in the first trimester when the pregnant woman is under stress. CRH levels rise throughout the second and the early part of the third trimester and then dramatically increase in the last six weeks. CRH regulates the duration of the pregnancy and fetal maturation. The amount of CRH in the woman's blood early in her pregnancy predicts the onset of labor months later.[6]

A few studies link prenatal stress to the higher risk of the baby developing allergies and asthma or having reduced immune function.[7] A subset of the full sample of mothers and children from the Children of the 90s study participated in an ancillary piece of research in which more than 5,800 families were monitored for eight years by Bristol University scientists. They found that the babies born to mothers who were very stressed during pregnancy were at a significantly greater risk of developing asthma.[8]

Prenatal Stress Does *Not* Have to Result in Problems

Despite the strong evidence of a connection between higher levels of prenatal stress and childhood problems, I want to again remind you that we are only talking about an increased risk of problems. Yet we are well beyond just "smoke"; now the "fire" is becoming obvious. Research is ongoing and we will continue to learn more in the coming years. We know that there are clear effects on the brains of the animal offspring of stressed mothers. Less clear is specifically how prenatal stress affects a human developing brain. The point to take home is that enough evidence now exists that makes it wise to take precautions where it is possible to do so. The steps necessary to reduce these risks are relatively easy to take.

Of course, events and situations that could cause distress are around all of us. We cannot avoid them no matter what we try to do. And it can be hard to gauge what a "normal" amount of stress is. How do we know when the stress we are under is too much stress?

The truth is that we all handle our tensions in different ways and we all experience different types of life problems. Many variables are involved in how much stress is too much for us and when that extra load on our nervous system will impact our child in the womb and beyond. In fact, some young women and their babies do not seem to be as affected by daily or even chronic pressures as others do.

That tells us something very important: *It is not the external events in and of themselves that are the problem.* If that's true, then identifying the baby's risk by whether a pregnant woman is undergoing "normal" or "abnormal" stress may not be the best way to go about diagnosing the problem. Instead, my best scientific and clinical intuition tells me that the most significant factors are these:

- How does your body respond to stressors?

- What is your baseline level of stress at the time you get pregnant?

- And how quickly can you reduce the negative effects of stress and anxiety on your body?

In other words, *I believe that the pregnant mother's ability to recover from variations in stress is what will determine the impact that any strain on her nervous system will have on her baby.* That's why I also believe that we need to and we can focus on prevention—how to help expecting women measure their stress levels and then rebalance their nervous system so they can reduce the possibility of problems for their babies. Before we move into the sections of the book that will show you how to do just that, the next chapter covers one last thing:

the dynamics of how too much stress on an expecting woman can cause potential problems in the womb.

This is a good time to take a relaxation break.

8

The Dynamics of
Prenatal Stress in the Womb

*When the mother is stressed, several biological changes
occur. . . . The fetus builds itself permanently to deal with this
kind of high-stress environment and once it's born may be
at greater risk for . . . stress-related pathologies.*
—Pathik Wadhwa, MD, PhD, University of California

Based on the evidence that we have reviewed so far, it's clear
that researchers are no longer asking if too much prenatal
stress can pose challenges for our children. At this point, researchers are trying to determine why it is true and how the
connection works. While studies link high levels of prenatal
stress to a variety of childhood problems, we don't yet know
exactly how the problems are triggered. The large follow-up
project I mentioned earlier, associated with the Children of
the 90s study and funded by the National Institutes of Health
(NIH), is, in part, an attempt to answer that question.

The mechanisms that scientists are proposing to explain
how prenatal anxiety can affect a child are complex and
include many factors and variables. As I noted earlier, it
likely takes not one but several of these factors converging
over a period of time to produce seriously negative effects

on the developing baby.

To understand the dynamics of stress in the womb, it's important to realize that the fetus and its brain are extremely responsive to their environment. A woman's emotions lead directly to hormonal and nervous system changes, which are then communicated to the baby's brain. As a baby is developing, its brain actually makes changes in its composition, structure, and functional characteristics based on its current circumstances. In this chapter, I've described some of the interesting research on this subject that has important implications for pregnant women. The endnotes describe some of the details of the research studies. Again, if you prefer not to explore the details of the research right now, you can return to the endnotes to read more later.

One Way Anxiety May Get Passed On

One prominent theory of how a pregnant woman's stress can affect her baby is the HPA axis dysregulation theory. If a pregnant woman experiences a lot of stress and anxiety during her pregnancy, she will likely have high levels of blood cortisol, which will circulate in the fetus. According to this theory, the brain of the fetus begins to consider the higher cortisol levels as "normal." It then decides that it does not need as many stress-hormone receptors in the emergent hippocampus (the hippocampus is the part of the brain that helps manage the stress response).

In effect, the baby's developing brain may reduce the number of cells that are meant to help the child deal with stress in the future. Chapter 3 described how stress hormones such as cortisol are produced when we face challenges or when we think, reason, or worry to solve a problem. Children who are born with a reduced number of hippocampal cells to help them cope with challenging situations have a hard time responding to upset since the cortisol remains in their system longer. Without the proper number of receptors to help the body eliminate the stress hormones, the child is more likely to experience anxiety and possibly depression. Simply put, *if a pregnant mother is chronically stressed, her child may become less able to handle stress.*[1]

Most of the research on how prenatal stress actually affects the developing brain has been done with animals. It has been harder to design studies with human infants; however, almost all of the scientists who have published on this subject agree that maternal stress affects the developing fetal brain through hormonal mechanisms, particularly through the interaction between the hypothalamus, adrenal cortex, and pituitary gland, or the HPA axis, which is activated when we are under stress. Activating this system regularly (chronically) eventually causes a dysregulation, or the loss of the ability of the system to work properly. In children whose mothers had stressful pregnancies or who experienced a higher degree of anxiety, HPA dysregulation in the mother has been associated with a child having greater emotionality and being difficult to calm down after a stressful situation. In other words, the HPA dysregulation is passed on to the child.[2]

More Stress, Reduced Uterine Blood Flow, Smaller Babies

Stress affects the flow of blood in our bodies, and that is another way stress can impact the growing baby. Each of us is sensitive to tension in a different part of our bodies. Some people feel it in the stomach, which causes them not to be able to digest their food well because the muscles in the stomach area tighten and restrict the digestive process. Other people feel tension in their heads and can even get migraine headaches from reduced blood flow during such periods.

A pregnant woman experiencing an overload of problems and worrisome thoughts may find that the blood flow in her uterus and placenta has been altered. Some studies have found that women who were the most anxious during pregnancy had significantly reduced blood flow through the arteries that feed the uterus. One possible reason for the abnormal blood flow pattern is that stress raises the level of hormones like noradrenalin and cortisol, which are known to constrict the blood vessels and decrease blood flow.

A study at the Queen Charlotte's and Chelsea Hospital in London investigated this issue. They found that pregnant women who scored higher on the stress questionnaires had "significantly abnormal patterns of blood flow through the uterine arteries."[3] Dr. Jean-Pierre Relier at the Hospital Port-Royal in Paris, France, did another study related to how stress can affect blood flow.[4] In his results, published in 2001, he reported that chronic anxiety caused increases in stillbirth rates and was linked to reduced birth weight. Dr. Relier related maternal stress to a reduced blood flow in the uterine arteries.

The issue of birth weight is important because small babies are more likely to develop coronary heart disease, diabetes, and depression in later life. Some studies looking at low birth weight found that the magnitude of the effects of stress and anxiety on birth weight was similar to the reduced birth weight found in children born to mothers who smoked.

A Woman's Emotional State
Quickly Affects the Baby

Fascinating preliminary work by Dr. Catherine Monk adds more information on how quickly changes in the pregnant mother's emotional status can affect the baby while still in the womb.[5] Dr. Monk's study used a clever design to demonstrate the differences in the babies' responses to their moms' distress. She compared the reactions of the babies in the womb of pregnant women who were chronically anxious and depressed *before* they ever became pregnant to the reactions of the fetuses of pregnant women who were *not* chronically anxious, stressed, or depressed before they became pregnant. Dr. Monk measured the babies' heart rates in the womb and the speed of their heart rate recovery after their mothers were experimentally "stressed" with a simple mental test. Even a simple challenge in the form of mental arithmetic or a task that requires attention and thought causes stress hormones to be produced.[6]

Dr. Monk found that the fetuses of women who had high anxiety *before* they became pregnant took longer to recover after their mothers finished the challenge test than the fetuses of women who were not chronically stressed before becoming pregnant. Dr. Monk concluded that if a woman with high anxiety becomes pregnant, her developing baby is likely to show stress reactions *even before it is born.*

Dr. Monk's findings are consistent with what has been expressed by many of the top researchers in this field—that over the course of a pregnancy, the fetus is exposed to and influenced by the environment in the womb. When this environment changes to include increased levels of stress hormones, alterations occur in the way the baby's brain develops, which may cause the child to be more susceptible to stress after he or she is born.

Stress Makes It Harder to Get Pregnant

Another way stress affects pregnancy through our hormones has to do with our ability to get pregnant. Dr. Sarah L. Berga has devoted her career to one of the most hotly debated subjects in the fertility business: getting pregnant without a lot of drugs. Dr. Berga is one of just a few doctors who is exploring how chronic anxiety may keep women from ovulating and how relaxation techniques may help. More precisely, Dr. Berga is looking at how chronic stress can change a woman's brain signals to the hypothalamus—the H in the HPA axis.

Her research suggests that a cascade of events, beginning with stress, leads to reduced levels of hormones critical for ovulation. Her research has also shown that women who do not ovulate have excessive levels of the stress hormone cortisol in their brain fluid. Dr. Berga's published studies generally include only a small sample of women, but the studies are very carefully done.[7]

What's Next?

From the perspective of both scientific research and public awareness, we are just now beginning to understand the problems caused by unmanaged prenatal stress. More research has already been planned to find answers to critical questions like these:

- What kinds of stress are the most damaging?

- How much stress does there have to be or how long does the stress have to last before we have to be concerned about it increasing the risk of harm to the unborn child?

- At what point does a constant environment of tension cause negative changes in the baby's developing brain?

- What are the most critical periods to avoid extra tension and challenge during pregnancy?

- Is the mother's tendency to be chronically stressed even before getting pregnant the real danger?

- Which of the possible relaxation techniques for pregnant women work best to prevent adverse effects on their children?

I could go on listing questions and issues that future research needs to embrace and answer. While this essential work continues, we can take what we already know about prenatal stress—and some simple solutions for it—and begin to act now to prevent potential problems.

What do you need to do to reduce your stress level before it gets too high? I've found that the best way to answer to that question is to first discover your personal baseline (or starting level) of stress and then determine how much additional stress is too much for you and will therefore tip you into the danger zone, where the risk of negative consequences increases.

Part Two will help you come up with those answers, which are different for each of us. You'll find a set of informal and easy-to-use rating scales to help you identify your baseline stress level, measure daily hassles, and then determine how much relaxation you need each day. And finally, in Part Three you can choose specific techniques—ones that best fit your personal tempo, preference, and style—to help you bring your system back into balance.

This is a good time to take a relaxation break.

PART TWO

The Stress Solutions
Formula

9

The A, B, Cs
of Stress Reduction

Here is Edward Bear, coming downstairs now, bump, bump, bump, on the back of his head, behind Christopher Robin. It is, as far as he knows, the only way of coming downstairs, but sometimes he feels that there really is another way, if only he could stop bumping for a moment and think of it.
—A. A. MILNE, *WINNIE-THE-POOH*

MOST OF US are like my friend Edward Bear. When the stress gets to be too much, we might not notice. If we do notice, we might say "rough day" and perhaps take some action to chill out. In general, though, we often just continue down the stairway in the same way, bumping our heads on every step. We don't realize how stressed we are until we overreact to some minor irritation or oversleep because we don't hear the alarm. I chose the quotation from *Winnie-the-Pooh* to open this chapter not only because Pooh was a childhood favorite of mine, but also because of the lesson we can all learn from that "silly old bear": if only we could stop bumping (stressing) for a moment, we might be able to think more clearly.

As you ponder what you now know about stress and what it can do, I think you will agree that it is time for a stress-reduction system that will work with our busy lifestyles. Here are the key points to keep in mind when looking for a good solution:

- It's not hard to trigger the release of cortisol in our body. Some people have a busy schedule and a busy mind, which leads to increased and possibly chronic levels of cortisol in their systems. Others do not have a busy schedule, but their busy mind never stops, and that definitely keeps a high level of cortisol in their body and brain.

- People today acknowledge that stress is affecting them more than it did in past years. Our lifestyle seems to generate stress because of our active minds and busy schedules.

- We know that when we are pregnant, we can ill afford to have high levels of cortisol remain in our system because that can potentially be damaging to our developing baby.

- While there are many stress-reduction techniques available in our arsenal, most people do not use them actively and regularly. Some may not use them at all, even though they recognize how stressed they are.

- One of the most effective ways to manage the problem of stress is to take frequent breaks during the day to stop the mental activity and consequent cortisol production.

All these points bring us to this logical conclusion: we need a simple and immediately available system that makes it easy to tell when we are stressed and then helps us get our stress levels under control. The system needs to be flexible enough to account for each day's special stresses and hassles.

In addition, it needs to take into account that each of us starts our pregnancy with a different baseline level of stress based on how our bodies have already been affected by the stresses in our lives. Some of us have lived with high cortisol levels long enough that our body has changed the way it deals with it. Others of us still have a body and nervous system that work the way nature intended it to work. Some of us live super-stressful lifestyles while others do not. Some of us have learned to moderate our daily activities to take regular little mental holidays or breaks in our thinking and work, and others of us have a hard time stopping our worrying and thinking or taking a break from what we are doing.

The bottom line: to be effective, a stress-reduction system needs to account for all these factors, and it needs to be a system you can work with not just by going to a yoga class after work if there is enough time left in your day. Instead, you need a system you can work with in the background all day long.

Taking all those factors into account, I have developed a stress-reduction system that is built around a simple formula and point system you can apply to your own personal situation. To better understand the formula, let's take a closer look at how a healthy nervous system works to automatically erase the effects of stress and cortisol and then look at what can upset that balance.

A Normal Nervous System
Works Like a Seesaw

The up-and-down action of a seesaw, or teeter-totter, is a good way to illustrate how a normal nervous system should work. *Going up* symbolizes moving into an active, working mode, such as when you are reacting to a challenge with a fight-or-flight response. *Going down* means you are relaxing and becoming less stressed. When we translate this model to our nervous system, *going up* is the action of the sympathetic nervous system and *going down* refers to the parasympathetic nervous system.

The autonomic (automatic) nervous system in our body works to manage stress in concert with the hypothalamic-pituitary-adrenal axis (HPA axis), which produces cortisol and other hormones to help you manage daily activities. The autonomic nervous system is divided into two parts: the sympathetic nervous system (stress reactor) and the parasympathetic nervous system (stress reducer). Their jobs are to balance each other, like balancing the two sides of the seesaw.

When the seesaw is evenly weighted or balanced, each side goes up and down with just a gentle push from each side. In the same way, when you think about dealing with stress in your life, you could think of it as doing a balancing act. Your goal is to keep the seesaw of life moving up and down within a range without getting out of balance too much or for too long.

Most of your body's systems have this built-in action ⇨ reverse-action because your body is designed to maintain balance (homeostasis). Your nervous system, in particular, is designed to work that way. Most people's nervous system immediately begins to rebalance the seesaw the minute it recognizes that the reason for being on alert is gone. As you get busy, excited, or involved in a task, your autonomic nervous system reacts by activating the sympathetic nervous system, allowing you to be ready to handle the activity or challenge. When your system is in sympathetic nervous system mode, you cannot fall asleep easily, digest food well, or empty your colon. All of those processes depend on the proper working of the parasympathetic nervous system.

As the work or aggravation of the moment is over, the other side of the seesaw—your parasympathetic nervous system—normally kicks in and starts reducing the effects of the sympathetic nervous system by reducing your heart rate, decreasing blood pressure, stimulating digestion, and saving energy. The action of the parasympathetic nervous system is vital to falling asleep, calming down from an anxious or fearful moment, and performing a host of other important body functions. The parasympathetic nervous system is designed to undo the effects that the stress has had on our body and mind. We might even stretch or yawn as a sign of relaxing. It's when our parasympathetic nervous system cannot keep up with the pressures placed on our nervous system that things can start to go awry.

What Goes Wrong: the Stress Tipping Point

In order to cope with our daily hassles and busy routine, our body secretes hormones—in particular, cortisol. When cortisol builds up and the sympathetic nervous system continues to be actively engaged for hours at a time (instead of the parasympathetic nervous system taking over to calm us down once the crisis is past), we increase the risk of damage when we are pregnant. Most of the research from chapters 6, 7, and 8 indicates that the increased risk of harm to the developing baby comes when the pregnant mom has too much cortisol in her system *for too long*. The more you push your nervous system by remaining in the sympathetic state of arousal, the more you increase the risk of your nervous system moving toward what I call *the stress tipping point*.

Your nervous system is trainable. Constant stress gradually trains and conditions your nervous system to respond in certain prelearned ways to similar types of situations. For instance, if your nervous system has learned to respond in a certain way to arguments with your parents or your spouse, your nervous system may start to gradually increase the speed at which cortisol is produced and your sympathetic nervous system will stay active longer. Over time, the parasympathetic nervous system loses its strength and the sympathetic nervous system begins to dominate. That is the stress tipping point.

The term *stress tipping point* as I'm using it here is not to be confused with the sociological concept of a tipping point into an epidemic of a disease or how trends are started and grab hold of the public mind, as described in Malcolm Gladwell's book *The Tipping Point: How Little Things Can Make a Big Difference*. It is also not to be confused with the normal ups and downs of a typical day. *The stress tipping point is the point at which your body begins to make a permanent change in the way it deals with stress.*

That change starts slowly. When we are young, most of us have a strong enough parasympathetic nervous system to be able to experience a fight-or-flight situation and then immediately begin the relaxation cycle. However, over time and with much worry, thinking, and emotional reaction, the parasympathetic nervous system gets weaker and weaker. As it does, the ability of our nervous system to easily rebalance itself—to keep the two sides of the seesaw in balance—can also weaken. When that happens, the sympathetic nervous system remains in control most of the time and we feel very little relief from the pressures of the day. Our nervous system stays on alert and we remain ready for fight or flight at a moment's notice. As a result, we may begin to have trouble falling asleep because it's more difficult to relax. We may even reach a point where it takes many days of vacation before we can begin to enjoy ourselves.

Reaching the stress tipping point does not happen overnight. The weakening of the parasympathetic nervous system is a gradual process that only happens to some people who feel very stressed for years and do not take time to relax and reduce that stress. Taking an annual vacation or even a couple of vacations a year while keeping a hugely busy schedule the rest of the time is not sufficient to avoid moving toward the stress tipping point.

When the sympathetic nervous system has dominated the parasympathetic nervous system for long periods of time (a condition called sympathetic distress), the changes in the natural balance of our nervous system can become permanent. At the stress tipping point, the body starts to show a large number of physical changes and even illnesses, such as insulin resistance and the metabolic syndrome, heart disease, digestion problems and irritable bowel syndrome, hypertension, insomnia, chronic fatigue, frequent colds, obesity, and even some cancers.

If we were to put the concept of the stress tipping point into our seesaw analogy, the picture would look like Fat Albert just sat down on the sympathetic end of your seesaw, and there you are, up in the air, struggling to get your parasympathetic end down. Fortunately, this severe situation is rare for most young people in their childbearing years. Research shows that it is hard to even get pregnant if you do not have a strong enough parasympathetic nervous system to help keep your nervous system in balance.[1] However, as is the case for many people today, it is not that rare for pregnant women to remain in sympathetic mode too often and for too long.

If you are in danger of reaching your stress tipping point while pregnant, you may not have started your pregnancy with a normal nervous system. There are many reasons this could be true, including genetics, childhood illnesses, and prenatal anxiety in your mother, to name a few. Don't despair if you are in this situation or are moving in that direction. It *is* possible to reduce your daily stress and get Fat Albert off your seesaw. Doing so requires conscious focus on daily relaxation, but it can be done, especially when you learn to keep in mind the factors that can prevent your nervous system from staying in balance. Table 4 lists a few of these key factors.

Paying Attention to How You Handle Stress

As I've been saying throughout this book, even if you have not reached your stress tipping point or don't consider yourself anxious, it's still very important to pay attention to how you handle stress. No matter what stress level you are at now, you'll stay healthier, and so will your baby, when you remain aware of how your nervous system—your seesaw—is functioning. As you can see from the list in table 4, in our increasingly busy life it's all too easy to slip into a stress mode, and stay there, without realizing it.

TABLE 4. Factors That Prevent Our Nervous System from Returning to Balance

1. Holding on to hurt feelings and anger
2. Thinking all the time
3. Worrying a lot
4. Resisting taking breaks while working
5. Feeling that there is never enough time to finish what you want to do
6. Feeling that you have too much to do

You'll notice from scanning the list that many of the factors that keep us in sympathetic distress are things that we do *with and in our minds*. This tells us that, for the most part, the real stresses that cause negative consequences originate in our minds and in our mental habits. While it's not easy to change your habits or your temperament, you can take the first step by being more aware of whether these factors are influencing your day.

When you recognize that you have been actively working and are in sympathetic (stress reactor) mode for, let's say, almost an hour, it's a good idea to disengage from your work and engage your preferred ways of getting back into balance. That might mean taking a few minutes to do some breathing, sing or hum to yourself, or listen to some relaxing music. Part Three offers many different choices for you to explore. The key is to space your relaxation breaks throughout your day. Sometimes simply changing what you are doing from a thinking mode to something you can do without thinking—like watering the plants, folding clothes, tidying your desk, or walking down the hall to deliver a folder—works well as a break.

This is a good time to take a relaxation break.

The Stress Solutions Formula

Now it's time to apply all the concepts you've been learning so far so you can personally work with the Stress Solutions Formula. Remember, I created this system as an effective and easy-to-use way to manage stress. Once you understand how it works, you'll see that it's not hard to put into action.

The formula for successful stress reduction:

A (baseline stress level) + B (daily hassles) – 25
= C (needed relaxation points)

In the seesaw analogy, A and B are on one end of the seesaw and C is on the other end. The idea is to try to keep things balanced and the seesaw working smoothly.

The Stress Solutions Formula will help you make managing daily stresses easier than ever because it incorporates a measuring stick—like a thermometer or stress meter, if you will—so you can determine when you are reaching the point where you need to take some steps to get back into balance. The numbers you enter into the formula for A and B will come directly from your answers to two questionnaires I designed, which you'll have an opportunity to complete on the coming pages.

The first questionnaire measures your baseline stress level (A) and the second measures your daily hassles (B). These are self-help questionnaires and, as such, are not standardized measures. In other words, they have not been administered to large numbers of people with specific levels of stress. I've designed these tools with what psychologists call "face validity"—that is, the items ask you about symptoms that most people clearly recognize as being related to chronic worry and anxiety.

Components of the Stress Solutions Formula

A = baseline stress level. The Baseline Stress Level Scale (A) measures how much your body is already reacting to its stress load by considering how easily you relax, how well you sleep, how much you worry, how active a thinker you are, and some common physical signs of stress. In effect, your baseline stress level shows how the stresses you've already experienced in your life are affecting you.

B = daily hassles. The Daily Hassles Worksheet is a simple checklist of many stress-producing situations. Your daily hassles score will change all day long as one stress ends and another begins, as one overlaps onto another, or as several are happening at once. Since the daily hassles score changes hourly and daily, it is important to have a blank worksheet on hand to keep track of your hassles as the day progresses. Or you can download our new Stress Solutions app to your smart phone or iPad.

C = relaxation points needed. To calculate the number of relaxation points you must earn in order to end the day in a generally more relaxed state, you simply take your baseline stress level score (A) and add it to your daily hassles score (B) and then subtract 25 points. Since we all have some stress in our lives—we all have to think and do things—I've assigned the number 25 as a constant that you subtract from A + B to come up with the number of stress points that you need to eliminate *on that particular day.* The Relaxation Credit Worksheet (C) lists various techniques and exercises you can use to relax and helps you add up your earned relaxation points.

Six Factors That Can Affect
Your Baseline Stress Level (A)

Your body is like a book into which a record has been made of how much stress you have so far experienced in your lifetime. Your baseline stress level (A) is an accounting of how much your body is already reacting to the daily or chronic stress you experienced *before* you became pregnant. That score is not likely to change much and it surely will not change quickly or from day to day. There are many variables that determine if you are on a path where you are likely to reach the stress tipping point in your lifetime. Here are six key factors to keep in mind that can increase (or decrease) your baseline stress level score.

1. The first factor that influences your baseline stress level is *how quickly and easily your system rebalances itself* after a rough day or an experience that puts you into sympathetic distress. In other words, does your nervous system automatically or easily return to a state of balance, relaxation, and

harmony? For example, I have a patient who tells me that when he takes a family vacation, by the end of the first week he is just beginning to feel relaxed and not quite as uptight. It takes him nearly seven days to unwind and begin to enjoy his vacation because his ability to relax is so impaired. Unfortunately, many vacations may only last four or five days. His wife and children have been enjoying the trip all along, but he cannot mellow out. He can't stop thinking about his work several times or more during the day even though he's away from work.

2. A second key factor is your *emotional reactivity*. Emotional reactivity is a term that relates to the degree to which you react to something emotionally and how quickly that happens. The higher your reactivity, the shorter your fuse and the more quickly you might enter a danger zone where your nervous system essentially remains in distress mode long after the stress or challenge is over. Some of us get upset simply standing in a long line to check out at a store. Others of us can withstand a lot of frustration before we get angry. And others can remain calm and levelheaded even in a crisis. A certain amount of emotional reactivity is, of course, necessary. If you never get emotional, that would mean that you would never get angry or passionate or happy. Anger can be helpful and it is important to be able to express our feelings, both positive and negative. What becomes a problem for your baseline stress level is when you are not able to let go of your negative feelings after you have become angry. Continuing to go over and over an event in your head is what raises your baseline stress level.

3. A third important factor that can increase your baseline stress level has to do with the *average degree of stress present in*

**TABLE 5. Six Factors That Can Affect
Your Baseline Stress Level**

1. How quickly your system can relax and rebalance itself
2. How emotionally reactive you are
3. What degree of stress is present in your lifestyle
4. How aware you are of being in a stressed state
5. How high-strung or anxious you were before pregnancy
6. What major events (storms, deaths, etc.) happen during your pregnancy

your lifestyle and your to-do list. Some people have long to-do lists and never make it through their list in a week, let alone a day. They get upset with themselves every day because the day runs out before they are able to check everything off their lists. They are always busy. Others can be happy just "vegging out" and taking it easy. And, of course, there are many degrees in between. Having a long to-do list isn't a problem as long as you apply the remedy of taking breaks, de-stressing, and making sure you allow yourself to have days where your to-do list is short as well as some days where you don't have a to-do list at all.

4. A fourth factor that can raise your baseline stress level is *how aware you are of the emotional and physical states that indicate stress.* If you are not aware of how you are feeling, you may not be as effective in reducing the stress that is building up. When that's the case, you can stay stressed for too long without realizing it. This is key: you cannot undo something that you are not aware of.

5. The fifth factor is related to *how high-strung or anxious you were even before you got pregnant.* Over the years, most of us have met people who say that they have been uptight and stressed and have been worriers for as long as they can remember. Others tend to take things as they come and are basically easygoing. If your nervous system was chronically stressed when you became pregnant, you are at a higher risk of more easily reaching and maintaining a high level of cortisol, which is where the risks to your child are the greatest. Women's cortisol levels always go up during pregnancy and reach a high point in the last months before delivery. So if you start from a fairly stressed state before you get pregnant or if you have a high-stress lifestyle, managing your stress levels regularly is especially important.

6. The sixth factor is the *number of major events and traumas that impact you during your pregnancy.* These events are often beyond your control. However, once you realize the potential impact of such events, you can take steps to deal with the effects during the event if it lasts a long time as well as after the event is over, which will help both you and your baby.

Calculating Your Baseline Stress Level (A)

The questions in the Baseline Stress Level Scale (pages 111 to 112) will help you calculate your baseline stress level by asking about your behaviors, feelings, and ways of thinking. As you consider each of these factors, keep an open mind and do not assume what your final score will be. And be honest with yourself—you are the only one who will see how you score.

The 25-item questionnaire is composed of five items in each of the five following areas:

1. Taking time to relax

2. Worrying or fussing over things

3. Amount and quality of your sleep

4. Mental activity and self-talk

5. Signs of physical stress

You can answer each item as *never* (0 points), *some* (1 point), or *always* (2 points). The highest score is 50, which is a simple addition of all 25 items answered as *always*, or 2 points each. You'll learn more about how to interpret your score and apply the formula in chapter 10.

A. Baseline Stress Level Scale

Instructions: Rate each of the items below to reflect how you tended to behave most of the time before you became pregnant. Don't just write the answer based on a hypothetical bad day or a good day you might have had. Your score should give you a sense of your overall response to stress over the past couple of years. Think about each item in terms of 0 = never, 1 = some, or 2 = always. Circle the number that best represents how you would rate yourself for each statement.

1. Taking Time to Relax	never	some	always
I feel guilty about resting or taking time for myself.	0	1	2
When I decide to relax, it takes time to really feel relaxed.	0	1	2
It's rare for me to take a break during the day for relaxation.	0	1	2
I hate to be interrupted before I am finished with a task.	0	1	2
I feel I have more to do than I have time to do it.	0	1	2
		Total 1	_____

2. Worrying or Fussing about Things	never	some	always
I tend to think about all the bad things that can happen.	0	1	2
It is hard to get worries off my mind.	0	1	2
I am likely to go over and over things that upset me.	0	1	2
I can feel so overwhelmed that I am close to tears.	0	1	2
When things go wrong, I am easily irritated and emotional.	0	1	2
		Total 2	_____

3. Amount and Quality of Your Sleep

	never	some	always
I sleep less than 8 hours a night.	0	1	2
I fall asleep dead exhausted at night.	0	1	2
I have trouble falling asleep at night.	0	1	2
I wake up still tired.	0	1	2
Once I lay down, my mind starts to run, think, go.	0	1	2

Total 3 _____

4. Mental Activity and Self-Talk

	never	some	always
My mind wanders.	0	1	2
I talk inside my head while others are talking.	0	1	2
My mind restlessly moves from one thought to the next.	0	1	2
I feel a need to be thinking or creating something in my mind.	0	1	2
Even after a problem is resolved, I cannot drop it and go on.	0	1	2

Total 4 _____

5. Signs of Physical Stress

	never	some	always
I sigh frequently when feeling stressed.	0	1	2
I find myself holding my breath when I get tense.	0	1	2
I am easily startled by sudden, unexpected, or loud noises.	0	1	2
I carry a lot of tension in my body (eyes, shoulders, stomach, etc.).	0	1	2
I am so nervous that I bite my lip, chew nails, or shake.	0	1	2

Total 5 _____

BASELINE TOTAL A = 1 + 2 + 3 + 4 + 5 = _____

Becoming Familiar with Sources of Daily Stress

Now that you know your baseline stress level, the next step is to calculate your daily hassles (B) and add that figure to your baseline figure (A). Your "daily hassles" are the aggravations and challenges you've faced today, and they can come from many different sources. Some sources of stress or daily hassles are worse for your baby than others. The sources of stress most likely to lead to later problems as your child grows up are surprising. One might think that major catastrophes like 9/11, wars, or even the death of a parent would take top place. But the problems with the greatest potential to harm your developing baby are negative patterns in your close relationships and daily life that upset you or cause worry, anger, or sadness.[2]

These daily recurrent patterns are things that happen or that you fear will happen nearly every day. They can include situations like constant conflict and tension in the household, a bad argument with your partner, significant financial pressures, having to do a job you really do not like, or problems with coworkers. Such sources of daily stress fall into the category of *sustained or frequently occurring stress*. Sustained stress produces high levels of cortisol on a regular basis. Moreover, since these are the kinds of issues that people have trouble getting out of their minds, their cortisol levels are not easily reduced. Thus, ongoing problems in your close relationships offer more of a problem for the baby's developing brain and endocrine system than single short-lived events because your cortisol levels are likely to stay too high for too long.

Not everyone reacts to stressors with an immediate increase in cortisol. Just having a bill you cannot pay or having an argument with your spouse does not automatically cause you to produce excessive cortisol. Remember that your nervous system learns, adapts, and is trainable. How you think and feel about that bill determines how you react. If you are angry, agitated, and keep thinking about what you "should have said" and so on, then your cortisol level may remain too high for too long.

The best of circumstances is when an expectant mother's relationships with her partner, family, and close friends can offer good support and provide a buffer against the stress and anxiety that accompany all the changes in her body, her emotions, and her life.[3] In fact, the more emotional and social support your interpersonal relationships provide, typically the better the outcome of your pregnancy. When that support is missing, the expectant mom needs to pay particular attention to tallying up her daily hassles and reducing them.

The daily hassles list also includes situations that do not repeat or are not constantly present, like having a surprise big bill to pay, getting into a minor fender-bender with your car, or needing an extra helping hand because your pet or child is ill.

Another source of daily hassles can come from your job or career. You might be pregnant while you are still in school or trying to finish a degree. That can surely add stress to your life. You may be working and cannot afford to quit or you may be working and do not want to quit because you are building a career. Those are all potential sources of daily stress.

Other areas of daily stress that could cause your body to produce too much cortisol are pain and personal health issues. Some women start their pregnancy with backaches or physical conditions that become more and more uncomfortable or painful in the later days of pregnancy. Toward the end of the last trimester, many women complain that they do not get enough sleep and do not rest easily because of pain and feeling uncomfortable. Some of you may not have been good sleepers to begin with and the pregnancy just adds to the problem.

Calculating Your Daily Hassles (B)

Taking all the possible sources of stress I listed above into consideration, the Daily Hassles Worksheet (B) on the following pages will help you keep a record of each day's stresses so you can get a realistic picture of how much stress you have had to handle during the day. The reason this is so key is that one of the issues in counteracting the negative effects of stress is our tendency not to realize how stressed we may in fact be.

The worksheet's seven categories of daily hassles include interpersonal and time stresses, performance and work stresses, mental and physical symptoms of stress, and any emotional stress that is the result of a fear you may be facing. On this worksheet, you also rate each stress on the basis of how long the event lasts. The list of daily hassles includes 27 possible stress-producing situations plus three additional spaces for you to write in other problems that may arise during the day. The highest number you could assign each situation is 5. Thus, in a worst-case scenario, your score for the day would be 150. That is highly unlikely, of course, but it shows you how quickly your daily stress level can go up.

B. Daily Hassles Worksheet

Instructions: Think about your day today. Is anything causing you to be upset or worried? Are you working on a timeline? Is today one of those days that you have too many things on your to-do list? Check the list below and assign a value based on the duration of the aggravation or situation. If the situation or problem lasts an hour or less, assign a number value of 1. If it lasts for a few hours, give it a 3. If the situation lasts more than 3 hours, assign it a value of 5. If you are not experiencing a situation that is listed, leave it blank.

Scale: 1 hr or less = 1   2 or 3 hrs = 3   >3 hrs = 5

Interpersonal Stress
(fight, disagreement, feeling upset, etc.)

_____ Feeling aggravated or frustrated

_____ Feeling hurt or angry

_____ Feeling sad or tearful

_____ Feeling misunderstood or unappreciated

Time Stress
(busy, late, too little time, etc.)

_____ Got up late, in a rush

_____ Stuck in traffic

_____ Hit a roadblock (literally or figuratively)

_____ No time during day for breaks for relaxation

_____ Pushing yourself all day to get something finished

Performance Stress
(giving a talk, paper, presentation, party, etc.)

_____ Feeling nervous before, during, or after the event

_____ Thinking about the situation before or after

Work Stress
(too much to do, don't know how to do it, etc.)

____ Been on your feet

____ Feeling aggravated by your boss, coworkers, or tasks

____ Fearful of not meeting a deadline or too much to do today

____ Facing threat of reprimand, loss of job, major failure

Mental Stress

____ Worried about what you said or want to say to someone

____ Being self-critical or judging yourself for something

____ Mind is active, challenged, trying to solve problems

____ Worried that you will not get something you really want

Emergency and Physical Types of Stress

____ Had an accident (car or other)

____ Encountered a major weather problem

____ You or someone close to you is sick or worse

____ Pain in back, neck, or other part of your body

____ Poor sleep, tired all day

Fears and Threats

____ Financial problems of concern

____ Fear something bad will happen

____ Fear of harm or major loss

Other Situations or Aggravations

____ _____

____ _____

____ _____

B = TOTAL OF ALL STRESSES TODAY ____

If you add your baseline stress level (A) together with your daily stresses tally (B), how high does your score of A + B get? In the next chapter, we will discuss some examples and interpretations. Now, let's complete the formula.

Completing the Formula: How Many Relaxation Points Do You Need Today?

You have seen how to derive A and B in the stress-reduction formula: (A + B) – 25 = C. In order to calculate C (the number of relaxation points you need to end your day in a relaxed state), you would first add your baseline stress level score (A) to your daily hassles score (B) and then subtract 25. (As I noted earlier, the formula automatically subtracts 25 points to account for the fact that all of us have to deal with some stress in our lives and we all have to think and accomplish tasks.) Record the number you come up with for C at the top of the Relaxation Credit Worksheet, which you'll find at the end of this chapter on page 126.

As an example, if your baseline stress level is 35 and you had a moderately stressful day (earning 16 points under your daily hassles), then A (35) + B (16) = 51. When you subtract 25 from 51, the remainder is 26. In this example, you would need to earn 26 relaxation points (C) before the day is done to rebalance your nervous system.

On the Relaxation Credit Worksheet, you'll see a list of the stress-reduction techniques offered in the resource guide in Part Three of this book. Each of these easy-to-use techniques is worth a certain number of points. In part, the points are based on how quickly and effectively the technique is known to or estimated to reduce cortisol levels. There is a more detailed explanation of each technique in the Stress Solutions Resource Guide in Part Three.

Obviously, the resource guide could not possibly include every relaxation and stress-reduction technique known or yet to be developed. If things you do for relaxation are not listed on the Relaxation Credit Worksheet, use your best judgment to determine their point value and add those points to your worksheet. Feel free to adapt the formula and worksheet where you see fit.

Tallying Your Score at the End of the Day

To give yourself an idea of how well you're doing each day in managing your stress, use the Relaxation Credit Worksheet to tally up how much, if any, unrelieved stress you have at the end of the day. You'll see this formula at the bottom of the worksheet on page 127: C – D = UNRELIEVED STRESS AT THE END OF THE DAY. Simply add up how many relaxation points you've accumulated throughout the day as you've completed the various relaxation exercises you've chosen to do. That will give you D, or your total relaxation points earned. Subtract your total for D from C (the number of points you needed to earn to relieve your stress for the day) and you'll see your ending balance.

Here's how that would look using the above example: If you needed to earn 26 relaxation credits for the day as your number for C and you completed 26 points worth of relaxation exercises, your final stress score for the day would be 0. The goal, of course, is to end each day with a 0 or negative number. That is the ideal, but many of us will not be able to do that or will only be able to accomplish that some of the time. (For women with low and medium baseline scores, your left-over number for unrelieved stress may even be a negative number.)

If you do have a small amount of points left over at the end of the day for unrelieved stress, don't panic. The next day, just try to take it easy if possible or carve out some extra time for relaxation. If you repeatedly end the day with a high score for your unrelieved stress, consider making some changes to your schedule. You'll benefit yourself and your baby greatly by regularly adding more relaxation techniques to your daily routine so you can get that final number down as low as possible.

Take-Away Measures Section

The next pages are a take-away section you can use to make multiple copies of the questionnaires and worksheets for your regular use. You can also visit the website that I created, www.StressSolutionsForPregnantMoms.com, to download and then print out these questionnaires and worksheets, or you can download the Stress Solutions app for your smart phone. The formula requires three worksheets: (A) the Baseline Stress Level Scale, (B) the Daily Hassles Worksheet, and (C) the Relaxation Credit Worksheet. Other tracking aides, such as weekly and monthly charts to look at how much unreduced stress you have and how you are managing your stress over time, are also available to download from the website. I will add new exercises and resources there as I discover them. On my website you will also find a blog and community space, where I welcome you to share your own ideas with others.

*Please turn the page for
the Stress Solutions worksheets,
which you can duplicate for your use.*

A. Baseline Stress Level Scale

Instructions: Rate each of the items below to reflect how you tended to behave most of the time before you became pregnant. Don't just write the answer based on a hypothetical bad day or a good day you might have had. Your score should give you a sense of your overall response to stress over the past couple of years. Think about each item in terms of 0 = never, 1 = some, or 2 = always. Circle the number that best represents how you would rate yourself for each statement.

1. Taking Time to Relax	never	some	always
I feel guilty about resting or taking time for myself.	0	1	2
When I decide to relax, it takes time to really feel relaxed.	0	1	2
It's rare for me to take a break during the day for relaxation.	0	1	2
I hate to be interrupted before I am finished with a task.	0	1	2
I feel I have more to do than I have time to do it.	0	1	2
		Total 1	_____

2. Worrying or Fussing about Things	never	some	always
I tend to think about all the bad things that can happen.	0	1	2
It is hard to get worries off my mind.	0	1	2
I am likely to go over and over things that upset me.	0	1	2
I can feel so overwhelmed that I am close to tears.	0	1	2
When things go wrong, I am easily irritated and emotional.	0	1	2
		Total 2	_____

3. Amount and Quality of Your Sleep	never	some	always
I sleep less than 8 hours a night.	0	1	2
I fall asleep dead exhausted at night.	0	1	2
I have trouble falling asleep at night.	0	1	2
I wake up still tired.	0	1	2
Once I lay down, my mind starts to run, think, go.	0	1	2

Total 3 _____

4. Mental Activity and Self-Talk	never	some	always
My mind wanders.	0	1	2
I talk inside my head while others are talking.	0	1	2
My mind restlessly moves from one thought to the next.	0	1	2
I feel a need to be thinking or creating something in my mind.	0	1	2
Even after a problem is resolved, I cannot drop it and go on.	0	1	2

Total 4 _____

5. Signs of Physical Stress	never	some	always
I sigh frequently when feeling stressed.	0	1	2
I find myself holding my breath when I get tense.	0	1	2
I am easily startled by sudden, unexpected, or loud noises.	0	1	2
I carry a lot of tension in my body (eyes, shoulders, stomach, etc.).	0	1	2
I am so nervous that I bite my lip, chew nails, or shake.	0	1	2

Total 5 _____

BASELINE TOTAL A = 1 + 2 + 3 + 4 + 5 = _____

B. Daily Hassles Worksheet

Instructions: Think about your day today. Is anything causing you to be upset or worried? Are you working on a timeline? Is today one of those days that you have too many things on your to-do list? Check the list below and assign a value based on the duration of the aggravation or situation. If the situation or problem lasts an hour or less, assign a number value of 1. If it lasts for a few hours, give it a 3. If the situation lasts more than 3 hours, assign it a value of 5. If you are not experiencing a situation that is listed, leave it blank.

Scale: 1 hr or less = 1   2 or 3 hrs = 3   >3 hrs = 5

Interpersonal Stress
(fight, disagreement, feeling upset, etc.)

____ Feeling aggravated or frustrated

____ Feeling hurt or angry

____ Feeling sad or tearful

____ Feeling misunderstood or unappreciated

Time Stress
(busy, late, too little time, etc.)

____ Got up late, in a rush

____ Stuck in traffic

____ Hit a roadblock (literally or figuratively)

____ No time during day for breaks for relaxation

____ Pushing yourself all day to get something finished

Performance Stress
(giving a talk, paper, presentation, party, etc.)

____ Feeling nervous before, during, or after the event

____ Thinking about the situation before or after

Work Stress
(too much to do, don't know how to do it, etc.)

_____ Been on your feet

_____ Feeling aggravated by your boss, coworkers, or tasks

_____ Fearful of not meeting a deadline or too much to do today

_____ Facing threat of reprimand, loss of job, major failure

Mental Stress

_____ Worried about what you said or want to say to someone

_____ Being self-critical or judging yourself for something

_____ Mind is active, challenged, trying to solve problems

_____ Worried that you will not get something you really want

Emergency and Physical Types of Stress

_____ Had an accident (car or other)

_____ Encountered a major weather problem

_____ You or someone close to you is sick or worse

_____ Pain in back, neck, or other part of your body

_____ Poor sleep, tired all day

Fears and Threats

_____ Financial problems of concern

_____ Fear something bad will happen

_____ Fear of harm or major loss

Other Situations or Aggravations

____ _____

____ _____

____ _____

B = TOTAL OF ALL STRESSES TODAY _____

C. Relaxation Credit Worksheet

Date: _____

My Stress Solutions Formula for today:

(A ____ + B ____) – 25 = C ____ (relaxation points needed)

Breathing	Relaxation Points	Credit
Pursed-Lip Breathing Exercise	+1 pt/min	_____
Belly Breathing Exercise	+1 pt/min	_____
Focused Breathing Exercise	+1 pt/min	_____
RESPeRATE Device	+10 pts /20 mins	_____

Music		
Music in Background	+3 pts/30 mins	_____
Feet Up, Doing Something Else	+5 pts/30 mins	_____
Feet Up, Listening, Humming	+10 pts/30 mins	_____
Special Program for Pregnancy	+15 pts/30 mins	_____
Special Program for Pregnancy with Bone Conduction	+20 pts/30 mins	_____
Ototoning	+10 pts/20 mins	_____

Mental		
Prayer	+5 pts/10 mins	_____
Affirmations	+5 pts/10 mins	_____
Take a Mental Holiday	+1 pt/each time	_____
Safe Place Meditation	+5 pts/each time	_____
Relaxation Response Meditation	+10 pts/each time	_____
Check in with Yourself	+5 pts/each time	_____
Rainbow of Light	+5 pts/each time	_____

Physical		
Prenatal Exercises	+2 pts/10 mins	_____
Prenatal Yoga	+3 pts/10 mins	_____

Laughter Yoga	+20 pts/10 mins	_____
Chiropractic Adjustment for Pregnancy	+10 pts/adjustment	_____
Enjoy Nature	+5 pts/30 mins	_____
Exercise Routine	+2 pts/15 mins	_____

Biofeedback

StressErasure	+5 pts/10 mins	_____
emWave Personal Stress Reliever	+5 pts/10 mins	_____
Stress Thermometer/ Stress Card/Mood Card	+3 pts/10 mins	_____
GSR2 Biofeedback Relaxation System	+5 pts/10 mins	_____

Personal Pampering

Curl Up with a Good Book or Movie	+2 pts/60 mins	_____
Warm Bath	+3 pts/each time	_____
Herbal Tea Break	+5 pts/each time	_____
Power Nap	+10 pts/each time	_____
Sit Down and Put Up Your Feet	+2 pts/20 mins	_____
Sleep	+1 pt/60 mins	_____
Massage for Expecting Moms	+5 pts/30 mins	_____

Other Forms of Favorite Relaxation

_____	+5 pts/30 mins	_____
_____	+5 pts/30 mins	_____
_____	+5 pts/30 mins	_____

D = TOTAL RELAXATION POINTS EARNED _____

C _____ (relaxation points needed today)
−D _____ (relaxation points earned)
──────
= _____ **UNRELIEVED STRESS AT END OF THE DAY**

10

Applying the
Stress Solutions Formula

⌒ ⌒

*Take rest; a field that has rested
gives a bountiful crop.*
—Ovid

EVERY WOMAN IS different and starts her pregnancy with a
unique set of circumstances. If you are someone who has a
low number for your baseline stress level, you will probably
be able to manage occasional days with more stressful events
without having to be concerned about potential long-term
consequences. Some young women, however, have a higher
baseline of stress going into pregnancy.

Additionally, some women (and men too) were either
born with a rapid and strong reaction to stress or have developed such a response as a consequence of events in their
lives. Among other things, this means they quickly produce
a lot of cortisol and therefore have to pay special attention
to balancing their stress levels. The higher your baseline is
or the more stressful a lifestyle you lead, the more important
using the Stress Solutions Formula becomes. In this chapter,
you'll learn what the different baseline (A) numbers mean
and how to work with the Stress Solutions Formula and its

point system to get the best results. I've selected the cutoff numbers for mild, moderate, or high levels of baseline stress based on the number of symptoms a person exhibits.

As a reminder, here is the Stress Solutions Formula: A (baseline stress level) + B (daily hassles) − 25 = C (the number of relaxation points you need so that your nervous system is rebalanced by the end of each day). If you succeed in earning all the relaxation points you need in C, then your remaining amount of unrelieved stress at the end of the day should be 0. First, let's focus on how to interpret your score for A.

If Your Baseline Is Below 10 . . . or Low Stress

Most young women in their childbearing years do not have high levels of stress in their lives. If your baseline number came out below 10 on the Baseline Stress Level Scale (A), you are less likely to need to keep a close accounting of your daily hassles and stresses (B) during your pregnancy. Those of you with a low baseline may also find that the number of relaxation points you need each day (C) often turns out to be a negative number.

That does not mean, however, that you should ignore the issues of stress and cortisol and how they could potentially affect your unborn and developing child. If you are in the low-stress category, I suggest you check your levels a couple of times a week and on days that are particularly tough. To do that, go through the Daily Hassles Worksheet (B) and then plug your totals into the formula (A + B) − 25 = C.

If your score for C comes out above 0 or if you do have a stressful day, choose exercises in the Stress Solutions Resource Guide in Part Three that appeal to you and that will reduce your numbers so that your unrelieved stress score for the day (at the bottom of the Relaxation Credit Worksheet) gets down to 0. Since the research suggests that the third trimester is a particularly important time to keep your cortisol levels low, even if your baseline is below 10, I suggest that you take some actions to reduce your stress during that time. Working with more structured programs during the last three months of your pregnancy is like taking out additional insurance.

One other thing to be aware of is that you may find that your scores are lower than you actually feel. If you score under 10 on the Baseline Stress Level Scale (A), but your personal feeling is that you are more anxious or stressed than your score reflects, by all means listen to your mother's intuition and take more time to reduce your stress levels.

If Your Baseline Is 10 to 20 . . . or Moderate Stress

Unfortunately, not everyone has a low baseline of stress. Many women have to keep working while pregnant or choose to keep working or going to school because their career plans require it. That is wonderful as long as you keep in mind that balance is the key. Forewarned is forearmed. If you need to keep working or living at a fast pace, use the worksheets to measure your stress and to incorporate easy ways to keep your final daily score close to 0.

If your baseline numbers are between 10 and 20, you will greatly benefit by measuring your hassles with the Daily Hassles Worksheet (B). You can make a copy of that worksheet (pages 124 to 125) and laminate it or go to the website for this book and print out copies to use every day. By using this worksheet daily, you will naturally come to recognize when you need to counterbalance stress during the day. With practice, you can develop the healthy habit of immediately using one of the techniques out of the resource guide when you feel stress so that you will already have some stress-reduction credits by the end of the day. Even if you do get that proficient, it's still important to use the Daily Hassles Worksheet during the third trimester of your pregnancy as a reality check and to keep yourself honest. You may discover by the third trimester that this process has become second nature to you and that your overall baseline has actually improved.

If Your Baseline Is Above 20 to 25 . . . or High Stress

What if you are in the high range when you measure your baseline level? If you are starting out as high as 25 to 30, it's best if you adopt a careful program of stress reduction. The main precaution here is that if you're in this high-stress category, even small amounts of daily problems can easily increase your baby's risk factor without you realizing it.

Some of us are normally high-strung and anxious before we get pregnant. It's common sense to suggest that if you are in this category, you are even more susceptible to the effects of stress during your pregnancy. Remember the study by Dr. Monk described in chapter 8 where she found that mothers who had been chronically stressed, anxious, or depressed before pregnancy had children with more problems than did mothers who were not as stressed before pregnancy?

Being in the high-stress category should not cause you to be upset, however. The Baseline Stress Level Scale (A) is intended to help you see that if you're starting out with a high-stress level before pregnancy, you simply need to be more aware of your daily stress level and develop the healthy habit of responding to it.

Rather than adopting the attitude that you are "just busier

than most women," you'll feel better and help your child more by tailoring a stress-reduction plan to suit you. You might choose to do one or more of the formal programs that are recommended in Part Three or add the help of a friend or health-care professional into your process. Use a laminated copy of the Daily Hassles Worksheet (B) or go to the website and print out multiple copies to use every day. Check in with yourself during the day, pick one or two tools out of the resource guide, and use these strategies when you notice your mind wandering or when you recognize some of the physical symptoms of stress. Keep in mind that using this process will also help you develop skills that will improve the quality of your life even after you are pregnant.

What If You Cannot Avoid a High-Stress Day?

Some days at work seem destined to be hard. We know we are going to be stressed even before it happens because of the activities we've built into the day. Likewise, we usually know when a day of running errands or tackling something tough will require extra energy. If you cannot avoid a high-stress day, don't worry. In most cases, your body will make adjustments and help you reduce the excess cortisol. If that's not the case, you can turn to the resource guide for help.

When you know it's going to be one of those tough days, simply plan ahead for small breaks of 5 to 10 minutes each. At the very least, take those breaks when you go the ladies room throughout the day. No one can keep you from taking a few minutes for yourself during a visit to the ladies room. When you get into the restroom, even if it's in a public stall, stay for 5 to 10 minutes. Sit quietly or stand and hum a favorite song in your head, do breathing exercises or do some visualization exercises (such as the Rainbow Light exercise that you'll read about in Part Three). The important thing is to take those short breaks to either focus on your favorite song or achieve a quiet mind and more restful state.

When I was an intern at the VA Medical Center in New Orleans, all my days seemed stressful. A saving grace for me during that year was taking the time to do the Rainbow of Light exercise. Conducting psychology consults at the VA Medical Center in those days required spending a lot of time on the elevators going from floor to floor, and those elevators were amazingly slow. I made it my business to start the Rainbow of Light visualization when I pushed the elevator button. Other people on the elevator were busy and usually in no mood for small talk, so it didn't raise any eyebrows. I did this with my eyes open and fixed, staring ahead or down at the floor. I soon began to realize the added benefit of this exercise—you can't do this visualization and think or worry about other things you need to do at the same time. The visualization halts the process of worrying and obsessing.

If you cannot move your mental focus beyond the stress of a hard day, do the next best thing: plan a long, relaxing evening for yourself. You have earned it. You could, for example, listen to calming music, elevate your feet and legs, and even take a short nap when you first arrive home.

An Example of a Moderate to High-Stress Pregnancy

Now that you've reviewed the Stress Solutions Formula and some of the research on prenatal stress and have a better idea of the potential effects of stress on your unborn child, let's take a closer look at an example of someone who has a history of a moderate to high amount of baseline stress and is a worrier. After I have sketched out Janice's story, I'll fill in her answers on the three worksheets so you can see what someone like Janice could do to reduce her stress. Even though Janice is an imaginary example, she potentially represents many of us. Her story will help you understand how to use the Stress Solutions Formula as well as recognize the warning signs of too much prenatal stress—flash points that all of us can learn from.

Janice is a prime example of someone whose mind is always busy or active. She is constantly talking to herself. To put it another way, she is busy in her head all the time. I've found that many of us have this same tendency but aren't aware of it. Perhaps you'll recognize this overactive mind in yourself if I ask you this: *Do you hear yourself when you are talking or thinking? Do you talk to yourself (inside your head) while others are talking to you? Or are you likely to go over and over things that upset you?* If any of these situations is the case for you, and the constant talking or thinking in your head takes the form of worrying about this problem or that deadline, you are likely to generate more cortisol than someone who is, for example, humming or singing a song in their head.

Janice's Temperament and Pregnancy:

Janice is 29 and she is expecting her first baby. She and her husband have been married for eight years and have been trying to have a baby for four years. One of the fertility doctors Janice consulted two years ago said that one reason it was hard for her to get pregnant was that she had a lot of stress in her life and was anxious. Janice hadn't totally believed that.

"Sure, it's hard for me to relax," she thought to herself, "but isn't that true for everyone?"

Now that she's finally pregnant, Janice isn't thinking about that anymore. She is so excited and happy to be pregnant. She's in her fourth month of pregnancy and feels that she is doing well. Her OB/GYN is keeping track of her weight and Janice is beginning to notice little changes in her body daily. She only wishes that she didn't have to work and feel so tired at the end of the day—or have to worry about her boss.

During her morning drive to work each day, Janice glances at her watch frequently. The traffic on the interstate creeps along so slowly that she's afraid she's going to be late. Her boss always has his eye on the clock, and she has been late a lot since she became pregnant. Her boss knows she has a right to maternity leave once the baby comes, but he only grunts noncommittally whenever she mentions it. Janice feels that he is angry with her for getting pregnant; but since he won't talk about it, she feels that all she can do is stew about it. She knows she shouldn't take it so personally, but it upsets her.

As day turns into night, Janice is still uptight. She has always had a hard time relaxing. Janice has the kind of mind that does not like to shut down at the end of the day. It often takes her an hour or more at night for her mind to stop working and for her to actually get drowsy enough to fall asleep. She wishes she could simply lie down and drift off as soon as her head hits the pillow, like her husband can do. Instead, she lies awake at night, her mind racing as she goes back over the whole day—what her boss said or did not say to her, how he looked at her, the expression on his face when she dropped the coffee pot. She worries that he might replace her if she takes too long of a maternity leave or if she has to miss work because something is wrong with the baby.

Before she got married, Janice saw a counselor for the nervousness she felt when she was around her boss. The counselor told her that she needed to learn how to calm down and become quieter in her mind. He told her that she had a mild anxiety problem. He gave her some relaxation exercises, which she did regularly for a while, and she also committed to a regular exercise routine. She did feel better while she was working out and doing the relaxation exercises, but, despite her good intentions, Janice felt she was too busy to follow through and eventually dropped both of these from her daily routine. With the excitement of being pregnant, she forgot about them.

When the time for Janice's delivery came, her labor time was typical for a woman giving birth to her first child. The baby's Apgar scores were normal (the Agpar score is a measure taken by the doctors one minute after birth and five minutes later, providing a quick index of the health and neurological integrity of the newborn). Janice and the baby came home from the hospital in the normal amount of time and everything seemed fine.

Janice's Baby:

Janice and her husband named their baby Charles after her husband's father. Charlie was adorable but extra fussy. It was hard to get him to sleep. He would fuss for what seemed like hours before he finally dozed off for a short time. Charlie was so fussy that, although his father loved him, he didn't like being left alone to babysit his son because he was afraid that he might not be able to quiet the baby down if he started to cry. That put more pressure on Janice, who could have used some quality time for herself.

When Charlie was almost one, his parents and grandparents were proud of how early he walked. He was also beginning to show signs of communicating and developing early language. Charlie was still a poor sleeper, though, and tended to be very active now that he could get around a bit on his own. In fact, you really couldn't take your eyes off of him because he was likely to get into anything and everything. He didn't calm down easily after getting upset.

By the time Charlie was 18 months old, Janice's mother, a third-grade teacher, was already warning Janice that Charlie might have a problem with being too active—that he might be diagnosed as having attention deficit hyperactivity disorder (ADHD). At two-and-a-half years old, Charlie continued to be extremely active and restless and still had a problem sleeping. He was eventually diagnosed with ADHD.

Measuring Janice's Baseline Stress Levels:

So that you can get an idea of how someone like Janice scores on the Baseline Stress Level Scale (A), I've filled in her form on the following page, completing the questions to reflect her personality. Since Janice is an imaginary example, she doesn't get a chance to deny any of her problems to herself. That's something for you to be aware of. Denial can surely creep in when taking these tests because many of us don't like to admit our faults to ourselves and tend to underemphasize or downplay our difficulties.

A. Janice's Baseline Stress Level Scale

Instructions: Rate each of the items below to reflect how you tended to behave most of the time before you became pregnant. Don't just write the answer based on a hypothetical bad day or a good day you might have had. Your score should give you a sense of your overall response to stress over the past couple of years. Think about each item in terms of 0 = never, 1 = some, or 2 = always. Circle the number that best represents how you would rate yourself for each statement.

1. Taking Time to Relax	never	some	always
I feel guilty about resting or taking time for myself.	0	**(1)**	2
When I decide to relax, it takes time to really feel relaxed.	0	1	**(2)**
It's rare for me to take a break during the day for relaxation.	0	1	**(2)**
I hate to be interrupted before I am finished with a task.	**(0)**	1	2
I feel I have more to do than I have time to do it.	0	**(1)**	2
		Total 1	**6**

2. Worrying or Fussing about Things	never	some	always
I tend to think about all the bad things that can happen.	0	**(1)**	2
It is hard to get worries off my mind.	0	1	**(2)**
I am likely to go over and over things that upset me.	0	1	**(2)**
I can feel so overwhelmed that I am close to tears.	**(0)**	1	2
When things go wrong, I am easily irritated and emotional.	0	**(1)**	2
		Total 2	**6**

3. Amount and Quality of Your Sleep	never	some	always
I sleep less than 8 hours a night.	0	**(1)**	2
I fall asleep dead exhausted at night.	**(0)**	1	2
I have trouble falling asleep at night.	0	1	**(2)**
I wake up still tired.	**(0)**	1	2
Once I lay down, my mind starts to run, think, go.	0	1	**(2)**
		Total 3	**5**

4. Mental Activity and Self-Talk	never	some	always
My mind wanders.	**(0)**	1	2
I talk inside my head while others are talking.	0	**(1)**	2
My mind restlessly moves from one thought to the next.	0	1	**(2)**
I feel a need to be thinking or creating something in my mind.	**(0)**	1	2
Even after a problem is resolved, I cannot drop it and go on.	0	1	**(2)**
		Total 4	**5**

5. Signs of Physical Stress	never	some	always
I sigh frequently when feeling stressed.	**(0)**	1	2
I find myself holding my breath when I get tense.	**(0)**	1	2
I am easily startled by sudden, unexpected, or loud noises.	**(0)**	1	2
I carry a lot of tension in my body (eyes, shoulders, stomach, etc.).	**(0)**	1	2
I am so nervous that I bite my lip, chew nails, or shake.	**(0)**	1	2
		Total 5	**0**

BASELINE TOTAL A = 1 + 2 + 3 + 4 + 5 = _____
6 + 6 + 5 + 5 + 0 = 22

You can see from Janice's form below that her baseline score is 22, which is in the high range. Remember, the baseline score is not likely to change over the time that you are pregnant. It represents your history, reflecting the chronic changes in your body that take a long time to develop as well as your habitual ways of thinking that are resistant to change.

Here is a recap of the main points of Janice's story to show some of her stress symptoms and why she scored that high: Janice glances at her watch frequently, fretting over the morning traffic. She is *frequently worried* that her boss will get upset with her for being late again. The possibility of being late triggers *a chain of negative thoughts* about being pregnant and about her boss.

Janice *cannot let go of things easily and is always thinking or worrying about something.* Even though she has nothing to gain and a lot to lose from this kind of excessive mental cogitation, she cannot stop herself from stewing about her problems. She is unaware that this kind of thinking, where she allows her mind to run on and on, if not relieved, can create a buildup of cortisol in her system and thus potentially harm her child's ability to pay attention or deal with stress. Janice doesn't recognize that she often *talks to herself while others are talking to her* and that she is *likely to go over and over things that upset her.* Janice also doesn't realize that this mental habit is likely to be at the root of her *trouble falling asleep* easily.

Our mental habits—what we choose to let our mind do or not do—are at the heart of the matter. The truth is that a major cause of stress and cortisol production is, quite simply, the ever-active thinking mind. In reality, it doesn't take much to cause our system to produce cortisol. That is why in studies that examine the effects of stress, the only thing that has to be done to stress the experimental subjects is to ask them to write a five-minute speech or count by threes backwards. Thinking, worrying, mental activity—these are the key factors that drive up cortisol levels and keep them high instead of letting them come back down.

Like so many of us, Janice *does not believe herself to be unusually stressed*, even when the fertility doctor tells her that her nervousness may have been keeping her from getting pregnant. Janice sees a lot of other people who she believes are just as stressed as she is. She thinks she is perfectly normal and so are they. Again, most young women who lead busy lives, particularly those who are working professionals, do not see that they are bearing more than a normal amount of stress. To be clear, some women are capable of dealing remarkably well with a superbusy lifestyle. Their systems naturally start to reduce cortisol levels once the cause of the stress is gone. They also are able to relax easily because the sympathetic and parasympathetic nervous systems are in good balance. That's not the case for people like Janice.

Now that we have Janice's baseline score (A) of 22, let's look at how she scores on the Daily Hassles Worksheet (B) on the following pages. When an expectant mother's baseline score is as high as 22, it's essential for her to pay attention to her stress levels during the day.

B. Janice's Daily Hassles Worksheet

Instructions: Think about your day today. Is anything causing you to be upset or worried? Are you working on a timeline? Is today one of those days that you have too many things on your to-do list? Check the list below and assign a value based on the duration of the aggravation or situation. If the situation or problem lasts an hour or less, assign a number value of 1. If it lasts for a few hours, give it a 3. If the situation lasts more than 3 hours, assign it a value of 5. If you are not experiencing a situation that is listed, leave it blank.

Scale: 1 hr or less = 1   2 or 3 hrs = 3   >3 hrs = 5

Interpersonal Stress
(fight, disagreement, feeling upset, etc.)

__3__ Feeling aggravated or frustrated

_____ Feeling hurt or angry

_____ Feeling sad or tearful

_____ Feeling misunderstood or unappreciated

Time Stress
(busy, late, too little time, etc.)

__3__ Got up late, in a rush

__3__ Stuck in traffic

_____ Hit a roadblock (literally or figuratively)

_____ No time during day for breaks for relaxation

_____ Pushing yourself all day to get something finished

Performance Stress
(giving a talk, paper, presentation, party, etc.)

_____ Feeling nervous before, during, or after the event

__5__ Thinking about the situation before or after

Work Stress
(too much to do, don't know how to do it, etc.)
____ Been on your feet

____ Feeling aggravated by your boss, coworkers, or tasks

____ Fearful of not meeting a deadline or too much to do today

__3__ Facing threat of reprimand, loss of job, major failure

Mental Stress
____ Worried about what you said or want to say to someone

____ Being self-critical or judging yourself for something

__5__ Mind is active, challenged, trying to solve problems

____ Worried that you will not get something you really want

Emergency and Physical Types of Stress
____ Had an accident (car or other)

____ Encountered a major weather problem

____ You or someone close to you is sick or worse

____ Pain in back, neck, or other part of your body

____ Poor sleep, tired all day

Fears and Threats
____ Financial problems of concern

____ Fear something bad will happen

____ Fear of harm or major loss

Other Situations or Aggravations

____ _____

____ _____

____ _____

B = TOTAL OF ALL STRESSES TODAY __22__

Tallying Up Janice's Daily Hassles

Based on a regular day at work, Janice's scores on the Daily Hassles Worksheet add up to an additional daily stress total of 22 points for B. Adding A + B (22 + 22) puts her at 44 points for the day. To complete the Stress Solutions Formula (A + B) − 25 = C so that we can see how much relaxation Janice needs for the day, we take her A + B total of 44 and then subtract the normal daily stress allowance of 25 points. That gives her a total of 19 for C.

Janice will be in sympathetic distress at the end of the day unless she takes steps to reduce that number. Since she knows that she has the kind of personality that will continue to work on a problem in her mind until she finally falls asleep, during the day Janice should ideally be looking for ways to reduce her stress and stop the cortisol from building up and staying high.

How Janice Reduces Stress—Is It Enough?

In our made-up example, let's say that Janice has not yet read this book and does not know about the dangers of prenatal stress and cortisol. She does not take any special measures to relax during or at the end of the day, though she naturally does a few things that help her to unwind. Let's see how much credit she gets from that without putting forth any conscious effort.

This is where we will use the Relaxation Credit Worksheet that was introduced at the end of chapter 9. As we've seen, Janice's high baseline starting point, plus her day's experiences and the way she thinks and holds onto things that are troubling her, means she ends up with an excess of 19 points for C in her formula. In other words, she needs 19 relaxation credit points to decrease the excess stress she accumulated on this day. If Janice earns 19 relaxation points, she will end the day at 0 with her nervous system in a more balanced state.

Now take a look at the Relaxation Credit Worksheet that I completed for Janice on the following pages. You'll see that without taking any special measures she earns 12 relaxation points. She listened to music while she cooked dinner for a half hour, earning 3 points. She watched a good movie for an hour and a half after dinner, which gave her a point for each half hour. Finally, the six hours she sleeps, though not ideal, give her 6 credit points. Without much effort, she erased 12 of the 19 excess points.

While these things did help lower her stress levels and Janice was more relaxed at the end of the day, she could have erased more of her stress if she had worked with the Stress Solutions Formula to calculate how many relaxation credits she actually needed. The critical point here is that Janice needed 7 more relaxation points to end this particular day with her nervous system in a more balanced state. In point of fact, someone like Janice is likely to have high levels of cortisol day after day if she doesn't intentionally work to reduce her stress, and those elevated stress levels put her unborn child at greater risk. The extra 7 points in our example is not the big offender; it's the buildup of stress that takes place over time.

C. Janice's Relaxation Credit Worksheet

Date: __**9-28-2012**__

My Stress Solutions Formula for today:

(A __**22**__ + B __**22**__) – 25 = C __**19**__ (relaxation points needed)

Breathing	Relaxation Points	Credit
Pursed-Lip Breathing Exercise	+1 pt/min	_____
Belly Breathing Exercise	+1 pt/min	_____
Focused Breathing Exercise	+1 pt/min	_____
RESPeRATE Device	+10 pts/20 mins	_____
Music		
Music in Background	+3 pts/30 mins	__**3**__
Feet Up, Doing Something Else	+5 pts/30 mins	_____
Feet Up, Listening, Humming	+10 pts/30 mins	_____
Special Program for Pregnancy	+15 pts/30 mins	_____
Special Program for Pregnancy with Bone Conduction	+20 pts/30 mins	_____
Ototoning	+10 pts/20 mins	_____
Mental		
Prayer	+5 pts/10 mins	_____
Affirmations	+5 pts/10 mins	_____
Take a Mental Holiday	+1 pt/each time	_____
Safe Place Meditation	+5 pts/each time	_____
Relaxation Response Meditation	+10 pts/each time	_____
Check in with Yourself	+5 pts/each time	_____
Rainbow of Light	+5 pts/each time	_____
Physical		
Prenatal Exercises	+2 pts/10 mins	_____
Prenatal Yoga	+3 pts/10 mins	_____

Laughter Yoga	+20 pts/10 mins	_____
Chiropractic Adjustment for Pregnancy	+10 pts/adjustment	_____
Enjoy Nature	+5 pts/30 mins	_____
Exercise Routine	+2 pts/15 mins	_____

Biofeedback

StressErasure	+5 pts/10 mins	_____
emWave Personal Stress Reliever	+5 pts/10 mins	_____
Stress Thermometer/ Stress Card/Mood Card	+3 pts/10 mins	_____
GSR2 Biofeedback Relaxation System	+5 pts/10 mins	_____

Personal Pampering

Curl Up with a Good Book or Movie	+2 pts/60 mins	**3**
Warm Bath	+3 pts/each time	_____
Herbal Tea Break	+5 pts/each time	_____
Power Nap	+10 pts/each time	_____
Sit Down and Put Up Your Feet	+2 pts/20 mins	**6**
Sleep	+1 pt/60 mins	_____
Massage for Expecting Moms	+5 pts/30 mins	_____

Other Forms of Favorite Relaxation

_____	+5 pts/30 mins	_____
_____	+5 pts/30 mins	_____
_____	+5 pts/30 mins	_____

D = TOTAL RELAXATION POINTS EARNED   **12**

C **19** (relaxation points needed today)

−D **12** (relaxation points earned)

= **7** UNRELIEVED STRESS AT END OF THE DAY

What Janice Could Have Done to Reduce Stress

If Janice had gone through the quick checklist of daily hassles, she might have realized that her stress was building and taken direct action during the day. To reduce her stress score further by the end of the day, Janice could have used any number of stress-reduction techniques that are described in Part Three of this book. For example, she could have had a cup of tea for 5 points, done a little breathing exercise for 5 minutes (5 points), and done the Rainbow of Light technique (5 points) to stop the mental chatter about the day as she lay down. Removing the last of her extra stress may have helped her get a better night's sleep.

Because of her tendency to have an active and worrying mind, Janice would have benefited most by using techniques that quickly reduce cortisol levels and quiet the mind. Most of the music techniques described in Part Three have unique cortisol-reducing abilities and can stop the mental chatter very quickly. You can see, then, from this example how useful the Stress Solutions Formula and Stress Solutions Resource Guide can be and how easy it is to integrate into your life.

Would Charlie have been less fussy, fallen asleep more easily, and been less apt to have ADHD if Janice had paid more attention to her daily stress levels during her pregnancy? We cannot know for sure because there are so many variables that play a role in a child's condition. However, we do know from the research to date that many common childhood behavioral issues, emotional problems, anxiety disorders, and developmental delays can result, at least in part, from too much unresolved anxiety and stress that the mother carries during her pregnancy.

That means that the probability (or risk) of Charlie having some problems would probably increase as Janice's stress levels increased. It could be that Janice would have given birth to a child with ADHD even if she had been careful to work on reducing her stress levels. Still, I believe that stress reduction is the best way we know of so far to decrease the risk for children potentially developing these serious problems. Said another way, by pregnant women making some changes to reduce their levels of stress, they can increase their children's chances of reaching their true potential.

Final Thoughts on Using the Formula and Point System

By using the set of measuring tools that are part of the Stress Solutions Formula, with its simple point system, you can take a lot of the guesswork out of trying to determine if and when you need to reduce your cortisol levels. Here are a few things to remember as you think about applying this formula in your own life.

Keeping a good balance between engaging your mind (which raises cortisol) and disengaging it (which lowers cortisol) seems to be a key issue for managing prenatal stress. Taking frequent breaks is also very important. There is a potential trap, though, that you need to be aware of: you can take a break in what you are doing and still be actively thinking or worrying or mentally active in some other way. That kind of a break will not help reduce your cortisol.

I realized as I was working on this book that taking a break from the computer did not mean that I was automatically stopping my thought process. In fact, sometimes my mental activity continued and became even stronger as I took a walk or prepared dinner. Some of us have a very hard time stopping our thought processes, particularly if we are trying to solve a problem or are worried about something. However, one thing that I know is true is that we are all capable of doing really tough things, things we might never do for ourselves, on behalf of those we love. Carrying a child, and knowing the impact we can have on that child's future, can give us the extra incentive we need to adopt a healthy habit of stress reduction, even if it takes a little effort.

Before we dive into the Stress Solutions Resource Guide in the next section of this book, where you will learn about many different and effective techniques to help reduce prenatal stress, let's explore in particular one powerful tool that can help anyone manage stress and anxiety: sound and music.

11

The Power of Sound
and Music for Relaxation

*Sound is everywhere—it is as much a part of our lives
as the air we breathe and the food we eat. But until now,
we haven't properly considered the health values of sound.*
—DON CAMPBELL & ALEX DOMAN, *HEALING AT THE SPEED OF SOUND*

MUSIC HAS PLAYED an important role in cultures around the
world. Common sense tells us that music can have profound
effects on human beings, both physically and emotionally.
Only in the last half of the twentieth century, however, has
music begun to attract scientific attention. In fact, the intentional use of sound and music for health-related applications
is a developing field that is composed of a large, collaborative
professional community, including medical professionals,
music therapists, musicians, psychologists, speech therapists,
educators, listening therapists, midwives, and other members
in the healing sciences.

This diverse group of professionals is collaborating on research that explores the intentional use of music and sound
for relaxation and health. The distinction between an intentional application as opposed to unintentional use of music
is the difference between having music on in the background,

where you may not notice it, versus sitting down and listening actively in order to relax and *intentionally* reduce your cortisol. Music, for instance, is now being used in hospitals and in operating rooms to stimulate healing. It is also making its way into the delivery room as well as into the daily routine for pregnant mothers all over the world.

Along with scientific interest in the benefits of music, there is increasing popular interest in self-help books about music, such as Don Campbell's best-selling book *The Mozart Effect*; his new book, *Healing at the Speed of Sound*, coauthored with Alex Doman; and *Musicophilia* by neurologist Oliver Sacks. As a result of popular books like these, more and more people are ready to embrace the positive and health-related benefits of music, and music is destined to play a more active role in the future of both medicine and education.

We have also seen a proliferation of toys, games, and do-it-yourself programs that brag that their product promotes smarter babies, brain growth, and even increased productivity. There is little evidence of effectiveness for many of these products. On the other hand, websites and articles written to debunk the wave of new products are also filled with misinformation and errors. While there has been more than a little consumer opportunism, we must not throw out the baby with the proverbial bath water.

A growing number of excellent music programs and CDs actually can help us relax and reduce cortisol. In fact, as I will shortly address, you do not need to do much more than give your attention to music in order for it to effectively reduce cortisol. In Part Three, the Stress Solutions Resource Guide, I have listed many references and web addresses for programs and people who offer sound and music resources of proven value. Some are even specially designed for pregnant women.

Among these is a program created by the Monroe Institute as part of their Hemi-Sync series called Opening the Way. Opening the Way is a program with information about pregnancy and delivery coupled with some meditation and relaxation sessions. Another great musical resource is the excellent Tomatis program for pregnant women. The Tomatis program for pregnant mothers is now packaged in a take-home format. Other music-based programs that are based on the work of the renowned French physician Dr. Alfred Tomatis include Drs. Kirk and Billie Thompson's EnListen (Sound Listening Corporation), Paul Madaule's Listening Fitness with the LiFT, and Alex Doman's The Listening Program (Advanced Brain Technologies). More information on these programs can be found in Part Three.

Humming and vocal toning are also tools for relaxation. These sounds are musical in nature and have the ability to soothe your mind, calm the nerves, and sometimes focus your attention. When people find themselves humming without consciously setting an intention to hum for a specific purpose, they are often filling time while doing something else that does not require their full attention. Generally, we hum when we are relaxed and enjoying our activity. You can also drown out that worried voice in your head by singing along with the radio or humming a favorite tune you know well. Humming, toning, and singing along with the radio or on your own are activities that are not only therapeutic but also free. You don't need any specific device; you are the instrument and you can do this anytime or at any place.

I've included the word *sound* in the title of this chapter because rhythmical and soothing sounds have been known for centuries to contribute to healing. Sound can be calming or it can be very irritating and completely destroy a peaceful mood. While all music is sound, not all sound is music. Many people live in areas where street noise can disturb their sleep. Purchasing a sound machine with a menu of sounds can be an economical option to help provide you with greater rest and deeper sleep. It can reduce the noise in your head if, like Janice, you have trouble falling asleep at night. The sound of the ocean, a babbling brook, the wind in the trees, and other sounds of nature are unequaled in their capacity to induce peacefulness and pure relaxation. The book *Healing at the Speed of Sound* offers many ideas for using music and sound in your everyday life.[1]

Early Discoveries That Music Can Reduce Anxiety

Some of the early research and musings on how music can reduce anxiety go back to the 1970s and 1980s. Joseph Chilton Pearce, noted author, lecturer, and visionary, talked about anxiety as a serious threat to society's children in his 1977 book *The Magical Child* and even described the music listening program for pregnant women developed in Paris by Dr. Alfred Tomatis (1920-2001). Dr. Tomatis, a French ear, nose, and throat physician, was a pioneer in the use of sound, voice, and music for healing.

I first learned about Dr. Tomatis and his work in 1991 and went to Paris to meet him. Through his work with pregnant women and music, Dr. Tomatis found a serendipitous solution to prenatal anxiety even before it was known to be a problem. In 1991, no one even knew the term prenatal anxiety, let alone realized that it could cause problems for unborn babies. Looking at Tomatis's important work in retrospect, though, it may turn out that his program helped pregnant women in so many ways because it reduced prenatal anxiety.

The Tomatis program for pregnant mothers is a music program to be used an hour to 90 minutes a day several times a week for up to 30 hours at the beginning of the third trimester of pregnancy. Mozart and Gregorian chants are listened to through a special tuner and headphones that have three speakers. Dr. Tomatis originally developed the electronic equipment that is used in this program.

The first study on the Tomatis program for pregnant women was conducted in two large general hospitals in the Paris suburbs in the early 1990s. Three groups totaling more than a thousand women were studied. One group of 245 women received the usual maternal care. Another group, consisting of 683 pregnant women, added breathing, relaxation, and birthing pool exercises to their usual maternal care. The third group, which included 223 women, added the Tomatis program for pregnant mothers to the usual maternity care, breathing, and relaxation exercises.

A large number of variables were studied, including a standardized, well-known measure of anxiety (the Hamilton Anxiety Scale), the method of delivery, the duration of labor, the state of the perineum, and the neurological condition of the newborn. Researchers found that in the group of pregnant women who engaged in the music program in addition to relaxation classes, there was a significant reduction in the time it took them to dilate before delivery.[2]

One of the most surprising and important findings was the outcome on the Hamilton Anxiety Scale, which the women took several times during pregnancy and after. Women who received no Tomatis program and no relaxation or breathing classes actually showed an *increase* in Hamilton Anxiety scores over their pregnancy. The group that used no Tomatis program but did take relaxation classes had a small decrease in anxiety on the Hamilton Anxiety Scale. Only the group of mothers who received the Tomatis program showed a very large decrease of 9.15 points in prenatal anxiety.

The Hamilton Anxiety Scale (HAS) consists of 14 items scored on a 5-point scale from 0 to 4, producing a range of 0 to 56 points. People with a generalized anxiety disorder or panic disorder usually score above 20. Those without anxiety will score very low on the HAS. Thus, a *decrease* of 9+ points is very significant and meaningful. Few other therapeutic methods have ever reported as substantial a reduction in anxiety.

Researchers concluded that there was no doubt that this form of music program during pregnancy reduced the level of anxiety of the women. The report of the study's findings also included a multitude of other measured benefits for both the mother and child. Considering what is now known about prenatal anxiety, many of those benefits are possibly related to a reduction in prenatal anxiety.[3]

In 2009, Dr. Wynand du Plessis, a clinical psychologist familiar with the Tomatis method for pregnant women, published a replication of the original Paris study in South Africa using two groups. Nine pregnant women in their third trimester spent 30 hours listening to a program of specially modified music of Mozart and Gregorian chants (the Tomatis group). Another group (the control group) consisted of 8 women who did whatever they would normally do for their pregnancy care.

The findings of this second study again showed significant reductions in anxiety, worry, and tension on several standardized measures among the women in the Tomatis group. The mothers-to-be in the Tomatis group also showed increases in satisfaction in life, motherliness, and agreeableness. In contrast, the women in the control group reported increases in tension and fatigue over the same period.

Anecdotal Evidence about Music for Pregnant Moms

Over the course of my career, I have had the opportunity to observe several dozen babies born to women who experienced a formal music-based program during their pregnancies. My daughter was 36 when she became pregnant. She was under a lot of stress during her second and third trimesters and I recommended that she add such a program when she carried my grandson. His delivery, though difficult, was probably easier than it would have otherwise been. Within a few hours after his birth, he showed the ability to move his eyes without moving his head and he made eye contact amazingly quickly for an infant.

In my office, I at one time offered the Tomatis Method, which uses modified music and active reading exercises to help children with certain types of problems. A young mother, Katherine, heard about this and brought her son, Jean-Pierre, in for evaluation and possible therapy. Jean-Pierre was six years old and had been diagnosed with auditory processing difficulties. When I first evaluated him, he was already struggling in school. I found out that Katherine had had two miscarriages before she became pregnant with Jean-Pierre.

Her pregnancy with Jean-Pierre had been difficult and she was put on bed rest for the last three months. Despite the best efforts of both Katherine and her physician, Jean-Pierre had been born three weeks premature.

I determined from evaluating Jean-Pierre that he could benefit from a listening program as a part of his regular therapy program. During the time that her son was doing the listening program, Katherine was again pregnant, beginning her last trimester. Understandably, she was worried about being able to carry to term. Katherine did not have a high level of anxiety in general. Her life, however, was very active and busy. Although she did not have a regular job, she was an active member of her small community, serving on many committees, clubs, and organizations. She participated in the PTA at her son's school and was always volunteering for local charity events. She confided to me that since her husband was a doctor in a small community, she felt obligated to be helpful to others. As a result of her feeling that she needed to show her involvement, it is likely that her cortisol level was often higher than it should have been and that she did not take enough time to relax.

While her son was working with his listening program, Katherine agreed to try the Tomatis program for pregnant women using the same equipment. She listened to her own 30-hour program for a period of six weeks. Katherine's OB/GYN was amazed that Katherine did not require bed rest with pregnancy number four and that she nearly carried her child to term. The baby, a girl, was born with no special issues. I saw Jean-Pierre for follow-up throughout his first four years of school and had the opportunity to observe his baby sister periodically during this time. Her demeanor was calm and she was a happy child, outgoing and social. After Jean-Pierre completed his work with us, I did not need to evaluate him again, but I did see Katherine a few years later at the grocery store and she reported that all was well with both children.

Most of the Tomatis-based music programs for pregnant mothers are now offered in the privacy of the listener's home. I no longer provide that service; however, I have personally observed that the children born to mothers who have worked with a formal music-based program while pregnant have a noticeably high level of emotional intelligence and a gentle and caring way with others. I have also noticed that they have an affinity for and seem to particularly enjoy music.

Another interesting bit of anecdotal evidence about the Tomatis program for pregnant women comes from actress Helena Bonham Carter, who played the evil Bellatrix Lestrange in the Harry Potter movies. Her story was featured on October 15, 2007 in an article in *The Daily Telegraph*, which reported that Helena Bonham Carter had used the Tomatis listening program while pregnant with her first son, Billy Ray.

Speaking of Helena's use of the Tomatis program, *The Daily Telegraph* article said: "During pregnancy, the technique is supposed to produce an alert, relaxed, and physically toned baby, and an easy delivery because it calms the mother. 'That was absolutely the case for me with Billy,' she says. 'Billy was able to hold his head up at a very early stage, he was very laid-back, and although I love chubby babies, Billy has always been physically toned. I really think listening therapy might have helped a lot. The birth wasn't drama-free, but I felt very relaxed.' "

Relaxing Music Can Reduce Cortisol Quickly

Apart from special programs that incorporate sound and music to help pregnant women relax, objective evidence clearly demonstrates that music alone, without the use of special equipment, has the power to calm and soothe the nervous system. In one of the first articles I found when looking at the connection between music and cortisol, Dr. Stéphanie Khalfa demonstrates that relaxing music quickly reduces cortisol levels. She found in one study that simply listening to music more quickly reduced cortisol than sitting quietly and trying to relax. Dr. Khalfa is a researcher at the French National Scientific Research Center in Marseilles, France. She was not looking for a solution to the problem of prenatal stress when she undertook that study, yet the implications of her results are key, as they reveal easy, affordable ways to reduce stress.[4]

Dr. Khalfa used salivary cortisol levels to monitor the level of a person's stress. Two groups of students were experimentally stressed by asking them to perform some simple tasks—give a short speech and do some mental calculations in front of an audience—both of which create enough stress to produce a measurable rise in salivary cortisol. The fact that such a small and seemingly harmless request can create significant amounts of measurable stress is, in itself, important. The two tasks actually create enough stress to make the increased cortisol levels last over a couple of hours.

Researchers were able to distinguish the effectiveness of different methods of reducing cortisol by measuring the drop or increase in salivary cortisol levels over time. After performing the two tasks designed to create stress, one group was instructed to listen to relaxing music that was audible in the room over a speaker system while they relaxed. The other group was told to sit and relax in silence. The results were significant: the students who were listening to music—as opposed to sitting in silence—showed an immediate reduction in cortisol.

The experiment revealed another surprising finding. The group of students who were relaxing in silence continued to show an increase in their salivary cortisol levels even after the stressful event was over. What happens in the person who is simply trying to relax in silence? Why do their salivary cortisol levels continue to increase for 30 minutes after the stressor has stopped? There's a good possibility that those who were sitting in silence were still thinking and continuing to stress themselves with their thoughts. On the other hand, the relaxing music may have helped to stop the wandering thoughts and allow the cortisol levels to begin to decline. In more technical terms, Dr. Khalfa and her colleagues reasoned that their study repeated findings of previous studies that showed that music is more effective than silence at decreasing the post-stress response of the hypothalamic-pituitary-adrenal axis.

The importance of this study cannot be overemphasized. The enormous value of being able to sit and listen to relaxing music and have our salivary cortisol levels immediately start to decline is impossible to calculate. In fact, the finding that music so rapidly and effortlessly reduces cortisol levels was a defining moment for me in deciding to write this book. If such a simple, easy-to-use, and effective tool to reduce cortisol were not immediately available, perhaps the argument of some researchers that we should not reveal a potential problem like prenatal stress without having a firm solution might have been more compelling. Yet, Dr. Khalfa's study and many others like it prove that there is at least one solution that is universally available for relatively little investment in time and money.

In 2008, researchers from the College of Nursing at Kaohsiung Medical University in Taiwan showed yet again how powerful a stress-reduction tool music is. They reported that listening to music alone, in the form of CDs, could make pregnant women less anxious and depressed.

The Taiwan study included 236 women with an average age of 30 who were in the last 18 to 34 weeks of pregnancy. The women were put into two groups, a music group (116 women) and a control group (120 women). The women in the music group were assigned to listen to music CDs that were 4 to 30 minutes long (lullabies, classical music, and na-ture sounds) with a tempo of 60 to 80 beats per minute (the same as a human heart). They were asked to listen to at least one CD every day for two weeks. The control group did not listen to any music. All the women in the study were tested on three measures of stress, anxiety, and depression before and after the music session. As in Dr. Khalfa's earlier study, the music had very positive benefits for the pregnant women who were in the music group. They were less depressed, less anxious, and less stressed than the other group of mothers. The study concluded that music provides a simple, cost-effective, and noninvasive way of reducing stress and anxiety during pregnancy.

You can see from the small sampling of research in this chapter that sound and music deserve a great deal of atten-tion as a stress solution because of their particularly potent and broad ability to help every expecting mother. Studying with Dr. Tomatis and seeing how much his unique program of sound and music helped pregnant women reduce anxiety is what began my exploration of prenatal stress. That was really the beginning of a 20-year journey that led me to write this book. The fact that Dr. Tomatis's special music program significantly helped pregnant women in a variety of ways led me to ask *"Why does it work?"* and *"How does it work?"*

Those questions, in turn, led me to take a closer look at the issue of prenatal stress and how it impacts both mother and child. What I found inspired me to develop the Stress Solutions Formula and compile the array of resources in the next section that are both easy to integrate into your daily routine and effective at reducing stress. It's time now to get familiar with the resource guide and see how you can use these tools to help you rest, relax, and stay in balance.

PART THREE

The Stress Solutions
Resource Guide

12

Creating Your Personal
Stress Solutions Plan

⬳ ⬳

The time to relax is when you don't have time for it.
—SYDNEY J. HARRIS

YOU ARE NOW ready to create your personal stress-reduction plan using the Stress Solutions Resource Guide to choose the techniques that will work for you. This part of the book provides many resource suggestions that you can use to earn the total number of relaxation hours you need each day.

We all have different likes and dislikes, habits, and needs, so having only one solution for reducing or managing stress would never work. By the same token, choosing just one stress-reduction technique (even a good one) for yourself during your pregnancy is simply not enough. This is particularly true for women who, before they are even pregnant, have a high baseline of stress.

The Stress Solutions Resource Guide allows you to pick and choose from a variety of effective techniques and exercises to develop your own individualized and safe program of stress reduction. The resources include a number of modern techniques and instrumentation as well as tools that date back to the early days of relaxation therapy and biofeedback, such as breathing techniques and the StressErasure device. The guide offers additional methods such as yoga, massage, and chiropractic care for expectant moms. While this book is geared toward helping pregnant women, anyone can use the techniques here to counteract the natural challenges we all experience.

The resource guide is not intended to include every known technique to reduce stress. These are suggestions. You'll also find some websites that can be a starting point for your own research into working with even more techniques to reduce your stress and cortisol levels. In addition, I invite you to visit my website at www.StressSolutionsForPregnantMoms.com, where you can read my blog, offer comments, and share your own favorite stress-reducing techniques.

The ways to reduce the effects of stress in this guide are intentionally as natural as possible. Keep in mind that this guide is in no way a substitute for following the advice of your physician. The techniques here are not meant to replace proper medical care. Always seek the care of a health professional when you are expecting. Be careful not to take supplements or health-store products to reduce cortisol while pregnant without your physician's approval.

Guidelines for Creating a Plan That Works for You

Let's quickly review the components of the Stress Reduction Formula: A (baseline stress level) + B (daily hassles) − 25 = C (relaxation points needed today). The Baseline Stress Level Scale (A) measures your body's reaction to stress prior to pregnancy. While your baseline score may change somewhat during pregnancy, it is the product of many years of your life. It will not change significantly in a short period of time or without sustained effort, and that's to be expected.

You will add your baseline stress level score (A) to the total of your daily hassles (B) to determine the number of relaxation credit points (C) you need to earn each day. Activities in the resource guide are assigned a numerical value that earns you relaxation credit for using them. I've assigned each technique a number of points based on its presumed or proven effectiveness in reducing cortisol and in raising your awareness of your level of prenatal stress.

The value for each activity is an estimate. An activity may have greater or lesser value for you based on how well you like it, how easy it is for you to do, how much the technique helps you become aware of stress, and how quickly it reduces the cortisol levels in your blood. Therefore, feel free to vary the amount of credit you assign to an activity by a point or two if you would like. The activities that you choose, the time of day, and the frequency with which you use them are entirely up to you. After you get an idea of what is available and what works well for you, I encourage you to mix, match, combine, and create techniques at will.

Here are five guidelines to help you put the resource guide's formula for successful stress reduction into action.

1. Develop a Habit of Checking How You Feel. Habits evolve over time with attention and repetition. Start with simply becoming more regular about checking in with yourself. Doing that at a specific time of day is a great way to develop a routine. Schedule one-minute "check-in breaks" three or four times a day to quickly assess how you feel—for example, when you go over your schedule for the day or get to the office, before lunch, at break time in the afternoon, and before bed. You can remind yourself to take these check-in breaks by setting reminders on your computer or smart phone or, if you are at home, set a simple kitchen timer.

You can also check in with yourself whenever you stop to take a restroom break or get a glass of water. On a particularly rough day, wearing even a loose rubber band around your wrist like a bracelet can act as a reminder to check how you are feeling. Whenever you look at your wrist, say to yourself, "Oh, yes, time to check my stress levels." In other words, set up ways to help remind yourself to become more aware of how you're feeling. All efforts you make to become more aware of how your body is handling problems will be positive for both you and your unborn baby.

2. Keep Track of How You Feel. When the alarm or ringer goes off or you look at that rubber band on your wrist, look at a copy of the Daily Hassles Worksheet (B) and run down it quickly, adding any points you may have accumulated since the last time you checked in with yourself. Don't be hesitant about adding points for stress. It is better to err on the side of caution than to deny stress and allow cortisol to build up. Keep a copy of the Daily Hassles Worksheet on hand and track your numbers on the sheet, in a small notebook, or on your calendar.

3. Choose Several Different Techniques That Appeal to You. Whatever category you are in (low, moderate, or high baseline stress), I encourage you to design a personalized program that suits your needs. The best antidote is to choose several different techniques that appeal to you and then commit to using them. After all, the methods are easy to use and the stakes are high.

4. Keep Track of the Stress-Reduction Actions You Take. You earn points when you *act* to reduce the stresses that accumulate throughout the day. During the day, see if you can find a few moments from time to time to do an activity from the resource guide. A small time-out to relax with one of these techniques will help you develop the habit of relaxing more and stressing less—and you will build up relaxation points so you won't have to do all your relaxing at the end of the day. As you go through the day, simply keep track of what you do to relieve stress. Jot a note to yourself or check it off right away on your Relaxation Credit Worksheet (C).

5. Get Familiar with How the Resource Guide Is Organized. The guide starts with a directory of solutions organized into categories. The activities, the number of points they are worth, and their overall value are listed for quick reference. The directory includes all the activities listed on the Relaxation Credit Worksheet (C). Following that, you will find an overview of each category (Breathing, Music, Mental, Physical, Biofeedback, and Personal Pampering) with a list of the suggested activities in each of the categories.

After each overview is a separate summary, or review page, providing more information for each individual technique or exercise. The summary page includes the following six key pieces of information.

Relaxation Credit Value appears at the top of each summary page. This is an estimate of how well that technique or exercise rates for relaxation. The number represents a value for the relative reduction of cortisol you can expect from using the technique. Each technique is assigned a number from 1 to 20 points; the higher the number of points assigned, the more quickly the technique is likely to reduce cortisol.

Next, you'll see the *Overview* of the technique or exercise with information about its benefits. The *Description* tells you how to do the exercise or technique. The section labeled *Other Ways to Use* gives an idea or two of how you can use this technique together with other resources in this guide.

If a purchase is involved, I've provided information on *Where to Find and Costs*. Many of the resources are free, but some resources to aid stress reduction can be purchased. In some cases, you can contact professionals or those who are specially trained in a technique to help you set up a program. This includes, for example, yoga instructors.

The Resource Guide Rating completes each entry. This rating uses from 1 to 5 baby rattles (🍼) to summarize the usefulness of the resource, with 5 being the most useful. The rattles function like the smiley faces or number of stars you see in magazines or on websites to give an overall rating to products. In this case, the number of rattles indicates an overall rating for effectiveness, ease of use, facility at reducing cortisol, and cost.

Final Words about Cortisol

Controlling your cortisol levels is important all through your life. However, the *most* critical time to control your cortisol levels is during pregnancy. As I've outlined in earlier chapters, elevated cortisol before pregnancy is associated with reduced fertility and lower conception rates. Part One of this book details the many conditions that are now being associated with high cortisol levels during pregnancy. After you deliver your child, elevated cortisol levels are associated with weight gain or an inability to lose pregnancy weight, increased appetite, sweet cravings, mood swings, depression, reduced sex drive, and suppressed immune system function (catching more colds).

The primary goal of the Stress Solutions Resource Guide is to help you reduce cortisol, and mental activity is what produces cortisol in the first place. Therefore, in order for any technique to work as an effective method of stress reduction, it must do three things: (1) stop the mind from its activity (thinking, worrying, ruminating), (2) reduce the levels of cortisol in your system, and (3) be easy and quick to use at least daily. Again, the points you earn and then subtract from your daily stress level total by doing these techniques will vary according to how fast and efficient the relaxation method is at reducing the cortisol.

Although no one knows all that is yet to be known about stress, and more is being learned all the time, this guide takes into consideration some of the key facts we already know about cortisol. In some cases, those facts may contradict what your intuition suggests. For example, physical overexercising can cause you to have *more* cortisol in your system instead of reducing it. Thus, if you are a runner or someone who spends a lot of time in the gym, you might be inadvertently creating more cortisol in your system. That's why you'll notice in this guide that you get fewer points for exercise than for other stress-reduction techniques that lower cortisol more quickly.

In creating the rating system, I've also taken into account another surprising fact—one that is as counterintuitive as the idea that hard exercise actually increases your cortisol.

Research shows that, sitting silently and relaxing may not be as quick and effective at reducing cortisol in our bodies as humming a song or listening to music.[1]

Remember, your personal stress solutions plan will work best when you tailor it to your own body, schedule, and preferences. What works for someone else may not work as well for you. So I invite you to experiment and explore, add and adjust—and most importantly, have fun—as you become more aware of how your body and mind respond to the various techniques.

13

What Can Dad Do?

Let's be a comfortable couple, and take care of each other!
. . . How glad we shall be that we have somebody we are fond of,
always to talk to and sit with! Let's be a comfortable couple!
—Charles Dickens, *Nicholas Nickleby*

A PREGNANT MOM rarely experiences her pregnancy alone. She almost always has someone in her life who cares and loves and wants to help, be it spouse, partner, lover, family member, friend, coworker, sibling, parent, or coach. This chapter is addressed to dads and those of you on a pregnant mom's all-important support team. If you do not have the time or the inclination to read this book cover to cover, you'll find suggestions here for specific sections you can read to learn why the pregnant woman in your life needs you and what you can do to help her reduce prenatal stress. By reviewing the main messages of this book, you will be in the best position to give her the support she needs.

Pregnancy and preparation for parenthood is a challenge for everyone involved as they are called to mature and respond to the changes in their lives. Expecting a baby can be very exciting when it is a planned event in a household with stable income and resources. Yet every situation comes with its own set of stressful circumstances, as much as we would like to hope otherwise. For a brief overview of how a pregnant woman's sustained high levels of stress can affect her baby, read chapter 6, "Landmark Studies on Pregnancy and Stress." It's foundational to understanding why it's so important to respond to prenatal stress with effective solutions.

While pregnancy is not completely about the mother, it can sometimes seem like it is to a spouse, partner, loved one, or coworker. No one likes to admit to feeling left out, afraid, or jealous; but as a loving support person, you may at times feel unappreciated, even though you want to be helpful. You may also feel that nothing you do to be caring is the right thing, especially when the expecting mother is having a particularly stressful and cranky day. Those are the times when you are called upon to be mature and when knowledge of what's taking place below the surface can put things into perspective. Many physical and hormonal changes accompany pregnancy, and most of them happen early on behind the scenes. So you can't tell what's happening just by looking. To gain some understanding of what those subtle changes are, read chapter 5, "The Body's Amazing Changes during Pregnancy."

Pregnancy is an extremely busy time for both parents. You can read chapter 3, "What Busy Schedules and Busy Minds Do to Us," to gain an appreciation of how stress affects all of us. Because stress is such a key factor during pregnancy, take particular care not to add to any tension or conflict. Keep arguments and criticisms to a minimum. The stress that is most damaging to a developing baby is ongoing argument and household conflict. Do little things to show the expectant mom in your life how much you love her and appreciate what she is going through.

Parenthood and the addition of another person in the household is a huge lifestyle change filled with new responsibility. Although it is exciting, it can also be a scary time for everyone. Change in and of itself can be stressful. Because of the dynamics of a pregnant woman's internal environment, including the delicate interplay of hormones in her body, she is more sensitive than ever to change and the stress it brings— and that stress can impact her more than it affects the rest of the unpregnant world. What's even more important is how the buildup of stress can affect the developing baby. Read chapter 8, "The Dynamics of Prenatal Stress in the Womb," to gain a better understanding of this.

Keeping Your Own Stress under Control

Keep in mind, too, that it's not only the pregnant mom who deals with more stress as the months go by. The nearer a woman gets to the main event, the harder it becomes for everyone involved. The third trimester is a very critical time, so use the first six months to prepare.

Learning to respond to stress is a healthy choice for everyone involved in a pregnancy. Many stressed women are, in fact, married to stressed men. Dad, while you may not think this book is about you, the more you take part in the process of helping your partner manage her stress, the easier it will be for all concerned. So I encourage dads as well as any pregnancy buddy, family member, or friend to use the stress solutions formula too. This could be one of the things that you do for the one you love. Learn what your own baseline stress level is in chapter 9 ("The A, B, Cs of Stress Reduction"), then review chapter 10 ("Applying the Stress Solutions Formula"), and finally choose relaxation techniques you like from the Stress Solutions Resource Guide in Part Three to ease your own daily stress.

Here are three important benefits for going the extra mile and putting forth the effort to follow these suggestions:

- Research is showing that mothers with lower stress levels have calmer babies. While I am not aware of any studies so far that prove that lower stress levels in a spouse or partner contribute to calmer babies, it makes sense that when there is greater peace, joy, assistance, cooperation, and love surrounding an expecting mother, she has a better chance of having a less stressful pregnancy.

- You will also benefit by using the Stress Solutions Formula and resources. Chapter 3 illustrates that learning how to better manage stress can improve general health and well-being, and that may very well improve the quality of your own life.

- Children learn by example. If either the parents or other participants in the pregnancy learn to manage their stress more effectively, that increases the chances that the growing child will learn those skills as well.

Your Role as Coach

If you are a father or partner of a pregnant woman or even her special friend or family member, think of yourself as a coach too. Coaching should go way beyond the delivery suite. After all, you are in the best position to know when your partner or friend is feeling stressed. You also know if she started the pregnancy with a high baseline stress level, as is true for many women with Type A personalities or with a history of worrying. You, better than anyone, know how she sleeps or if last night was a bad one.

Familiarize yourself with the tools and questionnaires in this book and then make it your job to coach her (or remind her, strongly but kindly) to take a break. As you are assisting your partner in keeping track of her daily stress numbers, you can keep track of your own as well. Together, you can review the various resources and decide which ones you want to try.

Coach her through the breathing and prenatal exercises. Join her in meditation and music. Be creative. Giving your partner a gentle massage can be a beautiful moment of intimacy. A Sunday walk in the park together or a bicycle ride in the beauty of nature is not only romantic but will also help you both unwind. Everything you do to support your loved one and to help her put the stress solutions into action will not only help her (and you) relax, but it can also boost your baby's potential to be a happier, healthier, and smarter child.

14

Directory of Resources

Breathing (pages 185–94)	Relaxation Points	Rating
Pursed-Lip Breathing Exercise	+1 pt/min	●●
Belly Breathing Exercise	+1 pt/min	●●
Focused Breathing Exercise	+1 pt/min	●●●
RESPeRATE Device	+10 pts/20 mins	●●●●●

Music (pages 195–210)		
Music in Background	+3 pts/30 mins	●●
Feet Up, Doing Something Else	+5 pts/30 mins	●●
Feet Up, Listening, Humming	+10 pts/30 mins	●●●
Special Program for Pregnancy	+15 pts/30 mins	●●●●●
Special Program for Pregnancy with Bone Conduction	+20 pts/30 mins	●●●●●●
Ototoning	+10 pts/20 mins	●●●

Mental (pages 211–25)		
Prayer	+5 pts/10 mins	●
Affirmations	+5 pts/10 mins	●
Take a Mental Holiday	+1 pt/each time	●●
Safe Place Meditation	+5 pts/each time	●●
Relaxation Response Meditation	+10 pts/each time	●●●
Check in with Yourself	+5 pts/each time	●●●
Rainbow of Light	+5 pts/each time	●●●

Physical (pages 226–40)

Prenatal Exercises	+2 pts/10 mins	
Prenatal Yoga	+3 pts/10 mins	
Laughter Yoga	+20 pts/10 mins	
Chiropractic Adjustment	+10 pts/adj	
Enjoy Nature	+5 pts/30 mins	
Exercise Routine	+2 pts/15 mins	

Biofeedback (pages 241–49)

StressErasure	+5 pts/10 mins	
emWave Personal Stress Reliever	+5 pts/10 mins	
Stress Thermometer/ Stress Card/Mood Card	+3 pts/10 mins	
GSR2 Biofeedback Relaxation System	+5 pts/10 mins	

Personal Pampering (pages 250–63)

Curl Up with a Good Book or Movie	+2 pts/60 mins	
Warm Bath	+3 pts/each time	
Herbal Tea Break	+5 pts/each time	
Power Nap	+10 pts/each time	
Sit Down and Put Up Your Feet	+2 pts/20 mins	
Sleep	+1 pt/60 mins	
Massage for Expecting Moms	+5 pts/30 mins	
Other Forms of Favorite Relaxation	+5 pts/30 mins	
_____	+5 pts/30 mins	
_____	+5 pts/30 mins	

OVERVIEW OF
BREATHING RESOURCES

BREATHING EXERCISES ARE at the root of relaxation as well as life itself. You don't even have to think to breathe. For this reason, breathing exercises are among my favorite ways to reduce anxiety. To do breathing exercises, you don't have to carry around more than you can handle. You can do them quickly throughout the day without interfering with your other activities. Breathing exercises can become a very natural part of your daily routine, and you can easily track when you do them so you can give yourself credit for them at the end of the day. Relaxed breathing can, in fact, be part of nearly all of the recommendations in the resource guide, but concentrating on your breath is an activity all its own.

Breathing connects you to and engages your parasympathetic nervous system as you take easy and rhythmic breaths. You will know that you have engaged your parasympathetic nervous system when you start to yawn. That signals the relaxation cycle and the rebalancing of the nervous system. Many people who are stressed find that they have a tendency to hold their breath at times, though they do not usually realize it. If you have a tendency to take a deep breath every once in a while, you are probably holding your breath.

Remember, during your pregnancy the changes in your body affect how you breathe. Because of those changes, by the time you are in your seventh or eighth month, you will be breathing 18 to 30 times per minute versus the normal 12 to 20 times per minute. Yet your oxygen consumption will only increase by 15 to 20 percent. So just being pregnant causes some physical stress as it takes more effort to breathe. The importance of this is that as your pregnancy advances, so does your physiological stress (because your breathing rate is increasing) and you may even experience a mild sense of struggle for a full breath.

On the following pages, I describe three breathing techniques along with one easy-to-use and not-that-expensive machine or device you can buy to help you relax more while doing measured breathing.

Breathing Resources

Pursed-Lip Breathing Exercise	+1 pt/min	
Belly Breathing Exercise	+1 pt/min	
Focused Breathing Exercise	+1 pt/min	
RESPeRATE Device	+10 pts/20 mins	

Pursed-Lip Breathing Exercise

Relaxation Credit Value: +1 point for each minute

Overview

The Pursed-Lip Breathing Exercise is an easy and very basic technique. It can be used anytime you feel stress build up, but it is best if you do it for at least 2 minutes (and up to 5 minutes) to really relax. Pursed-lip breathing is a good exercise to do during the day. If you cannot take a break to be by yourself, you can still do it right where you are and in the presence of others.

Description

Step 1: Prepare a place to do your breathing exercise. The key is to be comfortable and to be able to breathe easily. Usually the most comfortable position for this is laying flat on a pad on the floor or on your bed. Place a pillow or a rolled-up towel under your knees and neck to protect your lower back. If you can't do this, get into a comfortable sitting position.

Step 2: Close your eyes and become quiet. Breathe normally until you feel relaxed and ready to start.

Step 3: Begin to breathe in through your nose, then puff out your cheeks and slowly blow out your breath through lips that are slightly pressed together. You can accentuate this process by blowing out more slowly and for a longer amount of time until your lungs are almost empty. As you blow out the air, tighten your tummy, as this actually helps make room in your lungs so that you get a nice, deep inhalation for your next breath.

Other Ways to Use

1. Do while listening to music that is relaxing to you.

2. Can be done before or after other breathing exercises.

3. Add a visualization of releasing stress in some way while doing your breathing.

Where to Find and Costs

This exercise is free and available for you to do in your own home or wherever you are.

Resource Guide Rating

Belly Breathing Exercise

Relaxation Credit Value: +1 point for each minute

Overview

The Belly Breathing Exercise has many of the same positive benefits for reducing anxiety as the Pursed-Lip Breathing Exercise. Belly breathing is very helpful in reducing the stress of physical breathing and reduced oxygen consumption in the later months of pregnancy. Belly breathing helps you get a deep breath down to your belly, which gets more oxygen into your blood and makes you feel good.

As with all the breathing exercises included in this section, do the Belly Breathing Exercise in a focused manner and quietly for a period of at least 2 minutes and up to 5 minutes. Even better, you could do this or other breathing exercises several times a day for a few minutes. Belly Breathing is valued at +1 point for every minute.

Description

Step 1: Prepare a place to do your breathing exercise. It is important to be comfortable so you can breathe easily. Usually, the most comfortable position for this is lying flat on a pad on the floor or on your bed. Place a pillow or a rolled-up towel under your knees and neck to protect your lower back. You can also reduce stress on your lower back by bending your knees or by placing your legs and feet on a chair.

Step 2: Close your eyes and begin to notice how your breathing causes a natural rise and fall in your stomach.

Step 3: Place your hands comfortably on your stomach at the base of your rib cage. Take a slow, deep breath in through your nose so that your middle rises and gently spreads your fingers. Then quietly release the breath through your nose or mouth.

Other Ways to Use

1. Do while listening to calming music.

2. Can be done before or after other breathing exercises.

Where to Find and Costs

This exercise is free and available for you to do in your own home or wherever you are.

Resource Guide Rating

Focused Breathing Exercise

Relaxation Credit Value: +5 points for each 5 minutes
of breathing exercise or +1 point for each minute

Overview

The Focused Breathing Exercise is particularly designed
to relieve muscular pain and stress. You can easily tack this
exercise onto the end of the Pursed-Lip or Belly Breathing
Exercises. Like the Belly Breathing Exercise, Focused Breathing is very helpful in reducing the stress of physical breathing
and reduced oxygen consumption that can occur during later
months of pregnancy.

Focused Breathing is valued at +1 point for each minute
of practice. You could do this several times a day for a few
minutes at a time. Setting an alarm on your smart phone,
computer, or kitchen timer is a good way to remind yourself
to stop and take a breathing exercise break.

Description

Step 1: Prepare a place to do your breathing exercise. Get
comfortable so you are able to breathe easily. Usually, this is laying flat on a pad on the floor or the bed.
Place a pillow or a towel roll under your knees and
neck to protect your lower back. Or you can also reduce stress on your lower back by bending your knees
or by placing your legs and feet on a chair.

Step 2: Close your eyes and begin to pay attention to your
breathing and the natural rise and fall of your stomach. Continue until your breathing becomes easy and
rhythmic.

Step 3: Allow your mind to think about your body and find a place where your muscles are tight and need relaxing. Take a slow, deep breath in through the nose, while you are thinking about the tight muscles or area. Hold the breath for a count or 4 or 5, as you think about bringing lots of fresh oxygen to that area of your body.

Step 4: Quietly release the breath through your nose or mouth. Imagine the stress and tension melting away as fresh oxygen is carried by your bloodstream into the tight areas, making them more relaxed.

Other Ways to Use

1. Do while listening to music that is relaxing to you.

2. Can be done before or after other breathing exercises.

Where to Find and Costs

This exercise is free and available for you to do in your own home or wherever you are.

Resource Guide Rating

RESPeRATE Device

Relaxation Credit Value: +10 points for each 20 minutes of use

Overview

RESPeRATE is a device that was originally marketed as a method for reducing blood pressure. I have included it among breathing resources in this guide because RESPeRATE employs a system of inducing slow and regular breathing set in a rhythm with gentle tones (up for inhalation and down for exhalation). The net effect is extremely relaxing and has added physiological benefits for balancing the parasympathetic nervous system.

RESPeRATE is designed to be used daily or regularly in order to reduce your blood pressure. However, for stress reduction, it can be used anytime you wish, takes only 20 minutes a day, and is remarkably effective.

Description

When you use RESPeRATE, you will put on headphones and attach a breathing sensor (or elastic strap) around your chest. The device itself is about the size of a portable CD player. The headphones and sensor come with the machine.

Step 1: Sit comfortably and close your eyes. RESPeRATE's breathing sensor first analyzes your individual breathing pattern and then starts the program based on how you are breathing when you first turn on the unit.

Step 2: Simply listen to the melody through the headphones. The natural tendency of your body to follow external rhythms will enable you to easily synchronize your breathing to the tones.

Step 3: Gradually, the device will prolong the exhalation tone to slow your breathing. RESPeRATE slowly and comfortably takes you to the therapeutic zone of less than 10 breaths per minute. Once there, you will stay for a short period of time and then the program will finish. The entire process usually takes about 20 minutes.

Other Ways to Use

Use it daily or as needed for relaxation.

Where to Find and Costs

Prices start at about $299, but look for frequent special offers. Website information: www.resperate.com. RESPeRATE is now available at Rite Aid and many other pharmacies.

Resource Guide Rating

OVERVIEW OF
MUSIC RESOURCES

MUSIC CAN BE used in so many ways as an excellent antidote for prenatal stress and anxiety, ranging from using music from your own collection to purchasing specific selections that are reasonable in cost. Music is universally available, universally understood, and can be easily woven into the tapestry of everyone's life. In fact, you will see that music is or can be a part of almost every one of the techniques listed in the Stress Solutions Resource Guide.

Many music-based stress-reduction techniques are now available, and they are *not* all alike. This overview offers guidance on what to look for in your selection of a special program of music for pregnant women versus using music off the shelf.

Key Points to Remember: It's important to repeat two main points about the positive effects music can have on pregnant women. First, listening to music with no special gear or equipment has an amazing proven ability to quickly reduce cortisol. In chapter 11, I described a study that shows how quickly salivary cortisol decreases while listening to relaxing music. Second, listening programs that are especially designed for pregnant women and that use some special equipment—in particular, bone-conduction headphones—have been shown to dramatically reduce stress and prenatal anxiety.

Choice of Music: Your choice of music is important. Of course, taste in music is strongly personal, but classical music, waltzes, chants, easy-listening music, hymns, and lullabies are likely to bring relaxation the most quickly. I anticipate that someone will surely do a study soon comparing how quickly people show a reduction in salivary cortisol after listening to different types of music. I am doubtful that hard rock or rap will be the best choice for cortisol reduction, but I could be wrong, particularly for those who love that type of music.

The key to cortisol reduction is to listen to the music that helps you stop the self-talk in your head. A client with a severe anxiety condition once complained to me that the classical music she had listened to did not work that well to reduce her anxiety because she could still think over it. What worked better for her was music she could hum or sing along with. Songs that you can sing along with are likely to help reduce stress and your cortisol levels. If you are singing or humming along with music, you are probably less likely to be talking or thinking in your head.

CDs for Relaxation and Stress Reduction: Recordings (on CD or in other formats) that are designed for relaxation or for inducing a variety of different moods are plentiful. Many are even designed specifically to help pregnant women. Some of my recommendations are included in this resource guide, though there are many others to choose from. One or two of my recommendations offer music that has been trans-formed by way of sound engineering or the use of special headphones, an important aspect of the next group of formal listening programs for pregnant women.

Special Music Programs during Pregnancy: In addition to listening to recordings of music, you can also choose to work with one of the special music programs developed for pregnant moms. They vary in several ways. I have tried to organize the differences and similarities in such a way as to help you choose what's best for you. Some programs require special equipment, such as headphones with bone conduction, which you can rent or buy. Some can be done at home and some need to be done in a center.

Special Equipment for Bone Conduction to Buy or Rent: You can buy or rent equipment pieces that add a valuable therapeutic tool for stress reduction. The most important piece of equipment for anyone with moderate or high levels of baseline stress includes what is called bone conduction. Dr. Alfred Tomatis included bone conduction as part of his listening system by using a special vibrator or speaker in the headphones.

It has long been known that there are two inner ear mechanisms for hearing—air and bone conduction. While air conduction is by far the better known and understood of the two, bone conduction is equally important. Bone conduction in listening therapy systems especially helps those with a lot of anxiety and stress because it has the ability to directly influence the balance of your sympathetic nervous system (which reacts to stress) and your parasympathetic nervous system (which reduces stress) by strengthening the parasympathetic nervous system.

When you are in distress, it is usually due to your sympathetic nervous system overriding your parasympathetic nervous system, which I talked about in chapter 9. Bone conduction sends sound stimulation to the cerebellum and to the cranial nerves in the brain in such a way as to directly stimulate the vagus nerve, the tenth cranial nerve in the brain stem. The vagus nerve is a critical entry point into your parasympathetic nervous system. Stimulating your nervous system by using specially made headphones with a bone-conduction vibrator is a key to improving problems with sleep, digestion, and being able to relax. It also helps tone up your muscles and prepares your body for the rigors of birth and delivery.

There are only a few listening systems that offer bone conduction. The first was the Tomatis Method. Bone-conduction headphones are a primary part of that system. The Tomatis website lists trained consultants and practitioners who can deliver the Tomatis pregnant mother's program, called Preparation for Childbirth.

The only other listening system that specifically offers bone conduction along with a special program for pregnant moms is EnListen. EnListen offers the full Tomatis Method in a computer format.

Two other listening systems have added bone conduction to their equipment, but they do not advertise specific pregnancy programs. One, the LiFT (Listening Fitness Trainer) in Canada, is directly based on the Tomatis system. The other is from ABT (Advanced Brain Technologies). You'll find details and websites for all these programs on the following pages.

Music Resources

Music in Background	+3 pts/30 mins	
Feet Up, Doing Something Else	+5 pts/30 mins	
Feet Up, Listening, Humming	+10 pts/30 mins	
Special Program for Pregnancy	+15 pts/30 mins	
Special Program for Pregnancy with Bone Conduction	+20 pts/30 mins	
Ototoning	+10 pts/20 mins	

Music in Background

Relaxation Credit Value: +3 points for each 30 minutes

Overview

Background music is music from your collection or music you have purchased that you listen to in the background while doing something else, such as cooking dinner, reading a book, cleaning out a closet, and so on.

Description

Choose music that is relaxing as well as something that you enjoy, that makes you feel good, or that you can sing along with. It can be "elevator music," classical music, country, blues, jazz, or anything that appeals to you. This relaxation technique is worth 3 points for every 30 minutes that you listen.

Step 1: Play the music so that you can hear it while you work in the house, at your desk, or while you are doing some other activity. You don't need any special headphones or equipment.

Step 2: Listen for as long as you wish.

Other Ways to Use

Listening to music in the background while you are doing breathing exercises or mental exercises can be an added way to reduce stress. As long as your mind is not busy thinking, worrying, or scheming in any way, background music can help to reduce cortisol.

Where to Find and Costs

Listening to music in the background costs nothing extra if you already have the music on a CD, smart phone, or MP3 player.

Resource Guide Rating

Listening to Music with Your Feet Up While Doing Something Else

Relaxation Credit Value: +5 points for each 30 minutes

Overview

In the background-music technique on the previous page, you can be on your feet with music in the background. This relaxation technique is intended to be used sitting down with your feet elevated while you do something else. That something else can be anything from reading, playing a game on the computer, or playing solitaire to doing a crossword puzzle or watching TV or a movie. In other words, when you use this stress-reduction technique you are *not* mentally quiet, and that is why it is not worth more than 5 points per 30 minutes.

Whenever you are mentally active, you are necessarily putting some cortisol into your system. Yet the kind of relaxation in this exercise still reduces some stress and can be easier to fit into your schedule than some of the other techniques. You may also choose to listen to the music on a regular headphone or one that goes with your iPod or MP3 player. It is very easy to make your own playlist just for this purpose when you want to create a relaxing mood.

Description

Choose music that is peaceful and pleasing to you. Special instructions are hardly necessary as so much depends on what you are doing while you are listening to the music. The key here is that you have your feet up and are trying to take a few minutes to chill out.

Other Ways to Use

Playing music in the background while you take a power nap is great and can earn you extra points for the nap.

Where to Find and Costs

This technique for relaxing is as free as your choice of music and activity in your own room or house. While there are millions of musical choices available, the following sources along with your own Internet search can be potential starting points:

The Mozart Effect:

http://www.mozarteffect.com/

http://www.mozarteffect.com/OnlineStore/MERCPro
   ductb. php?id=6601

Advanced Brain Technologies:

http://www.advancedbrain.com/the-listening-program/
   the-listening-program.html

Monroe Institute:

http://www.monroeinstitute.org/program-list/

Resource Guide Rating

Listening to Music with Your Feet Up, Actively Listening, Humming, and Resting

Relaxation Credit Value: +10 points for each 30 minutes

Overview

The difference between this technique and the two before it is that in this situation, you are sitting quietly and actively listening to the music. You can be humming, singing, or just resting and listening while your eyes are closed.

Description

Again, choose your music so that it is relaxing. All you need to do is sit and actively listen, hum, or rest with your eyes closed. Be sure that you have your feet up and are trying to rest. Try listening to lullabies, hymns, or old favorites that you can hum or sing along with.

Other Ways to Use

1. A great addition to any music and relaxation program for expecting moms is to pick out some favorite children's books, such as *Winnie-the-Pooh*, *Le Petit Prince*, or Dr. Seuss books, and read them aloud to the baby in your womb while listening to music.

2. If you use the special music programs designed for pregnant mothers that incorporate bone conduction, you will earn twice as many points as you would by sitting quietly and listening to music because those programs add bone conduction.

Where to Find and Costs

This technique for relaxing by actively listening to music and resting is as free as your choice of music and can be done in your own room or house. If you want to do this with a special program of music for pregnant moms, see the next resource guide page. Here are some general sound and music resources to get you started:

http://www.sound-remedies.com/soundworklinks.html

http://www.mozarteffect.com/

http://www.apple.com/itunes/

http://spiritwinds.com/music/prenatal-music/

Or Google "relaxing music" or "music for pregnant women."

Resource Guide Rating

Listening to a Special Music Program for Pregnancy without Bone Conduction

～

Relaxation Credit Value: +15 points for each 30 minutes

Overview

The difference between this technique and the music relaxation techniques described on the previous pages is that this requires a program of music that has been specially selected for pregnancy. Unlike the category that follows, the kind of programs listed here do not include bone-conduction headphones. The programs in this category, based on the work of Dr. Alfred Tomatis, use music that has been specially modified to better stimulate your nervous system. Women who have a high baseline of stress can benefit greatly from using the programs for pregnant women with modified music because they are designed to be used over a certain period of time and for a certain number of hours a day. Choosing this kind of a program also helps you commit to using music regularly for stress reduction.

Description

Step 1: Settle yourself comfortably and put up your feet.

Step 2: Start playing the music (with a good headphone if so instructed). In general, no special equipment or special headphones are needed.

Step 3: While listening to the music, you can nap lightly, close your eyes, and rest, knit, crochet, draw, do puzzles, or simply do nothing. It really *is* okay to do nothing for 30 minutes or an hour!

Other Ways to Use

1. Read to your unborn baby while listening to the music.

2. If you are experiencing moderate to high levels of stress, you might consider a program with bone conduction (described next), as it helps your parasympathetic nervous system more quickly regain its balance and strength.

Where to Find and Costs

Costs vary depending on which technique you choose. Please consult the websites listed below for pricing.

EnListen for Expecting Moms:
http://enlisten.com/products/overview.shtml

EnListen programs for pregnant mothers that do not require bone conduction headphones are designed to be used by women who have low or moderate baseline levels of stress.

The Listening Program's iListen Basic Program:
http://thelisteningprogram.com/Getting_Started_
Program_Options_iListen.asp

The Monroe Institute's Opening the Way program:
http://www.hemi-sync.com/shopexd.asp?id=207

Opening the Way is a series of 8 tapes (also available as a digital download) with 14 exercises that include guided visualizations, relaxation exercises, information about a healthy pregnancy and the father's role, music for labor, breathing patterns for different points in your pregnancy, and other tools for after the birth. This program does not include bone conduction.

Resource Guide Rating

ᗯᗯᗯᗯ

Listening to a Special Music Program for Pregnancy with Bone Conduction

Relaxation Credit Value: +20 points for each 30 minutes

Overview

This music category includes programs for pregnant moms that use a special headset that delivers both air and bone conduction. Air conduction is how we normally hear. Bone conduction is perhaps the best way to reduce the effects of prenatal stress that have built up during the day. In addition to erasing the stress of the day (that is, reducing your anxiety and cortisol), the bone conduction adds a component of balancing your sympathetic and parasympathetic nervous systems and improving your muscle tone to make your delivery easier. These programs also use specially modified music, usually classical music. In addition, the equipment that plays the music further modifies it to enhance your attention and the effects on your nervous system.[1]

You may choose to listen for one 30-minute period a day or listen for up to one and a half hours a day. It is possible to skip a day here and there if you wish. The total length of the program varies and is not written in stone. The third trimester is a particularly good time to do the formal program with bone conduction, but the second trimester works as well. Women with high levels of anxiety should consider doing the formal program more than once during their pregnancy.

The music-listening programs with bone conduction listed here include those offered by consultants all over the world who are trained in the Tomatis, LiFT, and EnListen systems (EnListen offers a home unit for lease as well as a kit you can purchase for your own use). Many professionals have been trained in these techniques.

Description

Step 1: Settle yourself comfortably and put up your feet.

Step 2: Start playing the music with the special bone-conduction headphones.

Step 3: While listening to the music, you can nap lightly, close your eyes, and rest, knit, crochet, draw, do puzzles, or simply do nothing. It really is okay to do nothing for 30 minutes or an hour!

Other Ways to Use

Read to your unborn baby while listening to the music.

Where to Find and Costs

Costs vary depending on what you choose. Please consult the websites below for pricing and information for the Tomatis, EnListen, Listening Fitness Trainer (LiFT), and The Listening Program (TLP) systems, including the special headphones.

http://www.tomatis.com
   (click on the home page and then on "Find Us")

http://enlisten.com/

http://www.listeningfitness.com/index.html

http://thelisteningprogram.com/Getting_Started_
   Program_Options_BoneConduction.asp

Resource Guide Rating

🎧 🎧 🎧 🎧 🎧

Ototoning for Pregnant Women

Relaxation Credit Value: +10 points for each 20 minutes

Overview

Ototoning is a technique developed by Dorinne Davis, developer of the Davis Model of Sound Intervention. Davis discovered that not only does the voice produce what the ear hears, but the ear emits the same stressed frequencies as the voice. Likewise, when the ear receives the correcting frequencies, the voice regains stability.

Most people have heard of toning, typically with an "om" sound. Ototoning is more specific. Ototoning is accomplished by identifying the most important sound that the ear emits and then, through a special toning technique, toning that sound back into the body. The voice is used as the tool to make the change in each person. The ear provides the necessary tone or sound. For the pregnant mother, the sound will benefit both the baby and mother. Overall, Ototoning results in feeling more connected with your baby, feeling less anxiety, feeling more relaxed overall, and feeling more positive energy. This technique is simple and easy to use. Once learned, the technique can be used daily by the mother.

Description

The simplest way to start Ototoning is to use the Ototoner device, which produces the sound that you need to Ototone back to the body. Find a quiet place to sit on a chair with your eyes closed and feet flat on the floor. Your back should not be touching the back of the chair. The actual technique is described in depth in the book *The Cycle of Sound: A Missing Link and Its Healing Implications*. The Ototoning session should last at least 20 to 30 minutes to be effective.

Other Ways to Use

Ototoning can be done with or without the Ototoner device. See *The Cycle of Sound: A Missing Link and Its Healing Implications* for instructions.

Where to Find and Costs

Information about the Ototoner device can be found in *The Cycle of Sound: A Missing Link and Its Healing Implications,* available from New Pathways Press:

http://www.NewPathwaysPress.com/titlesforsale.html

To learn more about the Davis Center:

http://www.thedaviscenter.com/

Resource Guide Rating

OVERVIEW OF
MENTAL RESOURCES

THIS SET OF resources focuses on ways in which you can relax and reduce your stress using various mental exercises. These include affirmations and prayer as well as a number of simple visualization exercises that are designed to calm the emotions and quiet the mind. Remember, anything that will stop your thinking and let your mind be still will reduce your cortisol.

These techniques or exercises have long-term positive benefits in dealing with stress. Since they are generally slower to reduce cortisol than music and other techniques that can more quickly stop the mind from thinking, they may have a smaller relaxation value than some of the other exercises. On the other hand, you can do these mental exercises almost anywhere, without having to keep track of extra equipment.

Mental Resources

Prayer	+5 pts/10 mins	
Affirmations	+5 pts/10 mins	
Take a Mental Holiday	+1 pt/each time	
Safe Place Meditation	+5 pts/each time	
Relaxation Response Meditation	+10 pts/each time	
Check in with Yourself	+5 pts/each time	
Rainbow of Light	+5 pts/each time	

Prayer

Relaxation Credit Value: +5 points for each 10 minutes

Overview

Prayer can be a powerful means of reducing stress. For some people, simply turning over their problems to God and allowing themselves to be quiet is a great way to relax and become calm. If prayer works that way for you, great! If you are busy thinking and talking while you are praying, it may not reduce your cortisol levels as fast as music will. Needless to say, prayer has many other benefits too.

Description

Pray according to your own preference and tradition.

Other Ways to Use

1. Pray with quiet and gentle, rhythmic breathing.

2. Pray with appropriate music in the background.

Where to Find and Costs

No cost—just your time and love!

Resource Guide Rating

Affirmations

Relaxation Credit Value: +5 points for each 10 minutes

Overview

One way you can help yourself be your own coach is to use affirmations. Affirmations are positive, action-oriented statements that include the feeling you will have when you have achieved what you want. Affirmations help you focus your intention and reinforce the reason that you are doing an activity. They help you energize your time and actions with your attention.

Many people now use affirmations daily. Among the pioneers in the development of this mental exercise are Louise Hay, author of *Heal Your Body* and *You Can Heal Your Life*, and Dr. Wayne Dyer, author of *The Power of Intention*. There are many books and CDs designed to help you use affirmations. It is always a good idea to listen to and consider what you are saying in the affirmations before choosing which ones you want to use. By using affirmations, you are essentially feeding your subconscious a powerful statement, and you want to make sure it is the right message.

Description

Step 1: The best way to start to use affirmations is to get comfortable in a quiet place, usually sitting or lying down, close your eyes, and then repeat the affirmation several times. Always state your affirmations in the present tense.

Step 2: Think for a moment about what you are saying and what it means. Imagine that it has already happened. Let yourself feel what it would be like if what you are describing in your affirmation had already taken place. Here are a few examples of affirmations:

- This is easier than I thought.

- I am getting through this elegantly.

- I am dropping the stress of the day with every calming breath I take.

- I am feeding my baby peace and calm by doing these activities.

Other Ways to Use

Music is almost always a good accompaniment to saying affirmations, and some recordings of affirmations already include music.

Where to Find and Costs

There are many good resources to help you work with affirmations. You can create your own powerful affirmations or purchase books and CDs that will make suggestions and guide you through the process.

Resource Guide Rating

Take a Mental Holiday

Relaxation Credit Value: +1 point for each time
you take a mental holiday

Overview

This mental exercise helps you clear your mind and stop your
thoughts for a few moments. It is an especially valuable technique to use when you are in the midst of a busy day or when
you feel pushed to do a lot of things in a short period of time.
The trick is to stop your mental activity and imagine yourself
coasting or drifting aimlessly *in silence* for a few minutes or
even a minute. It takes practice, but the absence of words and
thinking is what makes this so effective.

Description

The goal of this exercise is to stop your mental processing. You
are taking a brief mental holiday as you stop your thoughts
and put your mind into neutral.

Simply take a deep breath, then mentally sit back, disengage, and let your mind coast or drift for a short period
of time. You can even imagine that you are disengaging the
gears of your mind, as if you are pushing in the clutch on a car.
As you go into neutral, let yourself stop thinking, processing,
problem solving, worrying, or whatever you were doing.

The more often you can remind yourself to slow down
and coast, the easier this technique will become and the more
benefit you'll get out of it. Try to remember to do this at least
in the morning and in the evening before bed. That is when
you can most easily find quiet time on a regular basis. When
you are having a very busy or stressful day, taking a mental
holiday a few times during the day can help you relieve the
tension that builds up.

Other Ways to Use

You can do this exercise with music or humming.

Where to Find and Costs

No costs and very little time are required for this technique of stress reduction. All it takes is some practice.

Resource Guide Rating

Safe Place Meditation

Relaxation Credit Value: +5 points for
each time you sit down to meditate

Overview

Over the years, researchers have studied the positive effects
of meditation on mind, body, and emotions. Meditation has
been proven to benefit breathing and blood pressure, calm
the mind, and relax the body. Of the many types of meditation
that exist, this guide presents only a couple very simple methods that are easy for any beginner to do. For the purposes of
reducing stress, I've put special emphasis on types of meditation that encourage calming or stopping your thoughts.

The Safe Place Meditation is the first of two easy-to-do
meditations in this guide. I encourage you to mold it into a
meditation that suits you best. The "safe place" is a place that
you can visualize in your mind's eye—a place where you feel
safe and at peace. It can be in a forest or a cave, by a mountain
or the seashore. It can be somewhere you have never been or
a place you remember as a child or visited as an adult.

Description

Step 1: Make yourself comfortable. Begin to visualize your
breath moving to key points on your body, known
as energy centers, as follows. With your first breath,
mentally direct the energy of your breath to your tail-
bone. Then, as you continue breathing, move your
focus and visualization to the energy centers in the
following locations: genitals, belly button, heart,
throat, forehead, and crown of your head. When you
release each breath, make a long, drawn-out exhaling
sound.

Step 2: Next, mentally count down from 5 to 4 to 3 to 2 to 1.

Step 3: Then, in your mind's eye, imagine a beautiful place in nature where you feel safe and secure. Imagine it at your favorite time of day. Imagine what it feels like. What is the temperature? What is the texture of the ground? Is it rocky or sandy or soft like a forest? Imagine what it sounds like. Can you hear the sounds of the ocean or the stream, the birds, the wind? Can you taste the place as you smell the air there? Is it a piney or salty smell?

Step 4: Here, in this place of safety and beauty, call in a guardian to be with you. This is someone you feel you can rely on—be it God, a guardian angel, a parent or grandparent or someone else, whether he or she is alive or not, real or not.

Step 5: Talk to this guardian about wanting a sense of peace and calm, about how you want your pregnancy to turn out, and how easy you want the delivery to be. Speak with him or her about any worry or concern that comes to mind.

Step 6: Imagine that person listening to you without saying a word. Say everything you need to at this moment. When you have nothing left to say, be still. Be quiet. Feel your guardian's reassurance, care, and love.

Step 7: When you are done, see yourself once again where you were at the beginning of your meditation—in that safe place. Feel your gratitude and then count yourself back to normal waking consciousness by counting from 1 to 5. Open your eyes and rejoin the everyday routine from which you just took a 10-minute to 15-minute vacation. Smile and feel refreshed and renewed.

Other Ways to Use

1. If you like this technique, you can record the steps and allow the recording to guide you through the meditation. This will make it easier for you to follow the steps and relax whenever you want to do this meditation.

2. Consider playing music that is calm and serene in the background.

Where to Find and Costs

No costs are involved in this using this technique.

Resource Guide Rating

Relaxation Response Meditation

Relaxation Credit Value: +10 points for
each time you do this meditation

Overview

This meditation technique is designed to calm or reduce your thoughts. Dr. Herbert Benson developed this technique and published it in 1975 in his book *The Relaxation Response*. It is based on a form of meditation called Transcendental Meditation, popular in the United States in the 1950s and 60s. This technique can be very powerful and bring many benefits if you do it regularly (once or twice a day for 10 to 20 minutes).

Description

The Relaxation Response Meditation requires that you focus on your breathing and use a simple word, such as *one*, to focus your attention. Dr. Benson's readily available book is the best way to fully learn the steps he recommends, and it doesn't take a lot of reading or practice to be able to do this technique.

Other Ways to Use

This meditation is meant to be used on its own.

Where to Find and Costs

You can purchase *The Relaxation Response* by Dr. Herbert Benson as a new or used book or borrow it from your local library. There are no other costs involved for you to use this effective technique. For a quick overview of the Relaxation Response technique, visit this web page:

http://www.relaxationresponse.org/steps/

Resource Guide Rating

Check in with Yourself

Relaxation Credit Value: +5 points
for each time you check in with yourself

Overview

It's a good idea to set up a daily ritual that helps you briefly check in with yourself to see how you feel. What you are primarily looking for is a way of improving your awareness of your stress levels and how your body is doing.

Description

Step 1: Take a few breaths. Try to clear your mind. It helps to close your eyes and block out any thoughts for a few seconds.

Step 2: Now focus on your body. Mentally scan your body. Visualize in your mind's eye each part of your body—starting at your feet and slowly working up toward your head—as you look for and sense any tight muscles, pain, or distress.

Step 3: If you find some bodily distress, use the Focused Breathing technique to reduce it. Here is a short version of the steps to that exercise for easy reference:

- Get comfortable.
- Close your eyes and pay attention to your breathing and the natural rise and fall of your stomach. Continue until your breathing becomes easy and rhythmic.
- Think about the place in your body that is in distress and needs relaxing. Take a slow, deep breath in through your nose while you are thinking about the tight muscles or distressed area. Hold your breath for a count of 4 or 5 as you think about bringing lots of fresh oxygen to that area of your body.

- Quietly release the breath through your nose or mouth as you imagine the stress and tension melting away.

Step 4: Breathing normally now, clear your mind and check in with how you are feeling emotionally.

Step 5: If you find that you have some thoughts and feelings that are sources of distress, estimate how much longer you will have to be occupied with them. Set a specific time when you will move on. For instance, tell yourself: "I'll work on _____ (for example, what I need to tell my boss) for 15 more minutes and then I'll take a rest before dinner." Or in your mind's eye simply encircle the sources of distress with a bubble of light and blow them away.

Step 6: If you can't set aside an issue or stop thinking about something on your own (say you can't stop thinking about a work project), then thumb through the resource guide until you find a technique you like that will help you stop your thinking. Examples of these include the music techniques, mental exercises like the Relaxation Response Meditation, reading a book, watching a movie, and other techniques.

Other Ways to Use

Use the Check-in-with-Yourself technique after you have completed the Take-a-Mental-Holiday exercise (page 215).

Where to Find and Costs

This technique only costs you time, and it works because it increases conscious awareness.

Resource Guide Rating

☕☕☕

Rainbow of Light

Relaxation Credit Value: +5 points for each time

Overview

Rainbow of Light is another mini-mental exercise that can have many variations. One of the benefits of this exercise is that it helps stop the process of worrying and obsessing because you are concentrating on visualizing.

Years ago, I adapted this exercise and used it multiple times a day during the year that I was in my clinical psychology internship at the VA hospital. VA hospitals are renowned for being stress producers due to miles of red tape. In New Orleans, that hospital was also the winner of my "Slowest and Least Reliable Elevator System" category. In order to reduce my stress while waiting at the elevators, I would practice this mini-mental exercise.

You can use this technique anytime you have a chance to wisely use your time to relax and get yourself back into a more peaceful rhythm, whether you're on a break, taking a moment to use the restroom, standing in line to check out at the grocery store, or waiting for the elevator to arrive at your floor. If you are in a crowd or on public transportation, you can easily do this visualization with your eyes open and no one need know what you are doing. It doesn't take long to use this technique; by the time you reach the last step of this visualization, the elevator (or whatever you are waiting for) is usually opening its doors.

Description

Step 1: Imagine a rainbow in your mind's eye, as if you were looking at one across the horizon. Then, starting with the red color of the light, see the light from that band of the rainbow enter the top of your head and travel swiftly down through your body, spine, and organ systems, exiting at your feet and traveling into the ground. Hold the intention that the light will take along with it all the stress and fatigue in your body and mind and deposit them deep into the earth.

Step 2: Repeat the process with orange light, then yellow, green, blue, purple, and finally white light.

Other Ways to Use

Do the Rainbow of Light technique even when you are not feeling extremely stressed as a way of preventing the buildup of tension in your body.

Where to Find and Costs

No costs are involved.

Resource Guide Rating

🍥🍥🍥

OVERVIEW OF
PHYSICAL RESOURCES

EXERCISE KEEPS OUR muscles and organ systems toned and operating well. Physical exercise can clear a cluttered mind and help sharpen your focus. Emotionally, it releases endorphins (brain chemicals) that relax you and help you feel good. If you want to begin a new aerobic program, consult your health-care provider first or try a program under the guidance of a trained professional. As long as your medical doctor agrees, if the exercise program that you followed before your pregnancy makes you feel good while you are doing it and afterward, then keep doing it.

Comfort is the most important principle of exercise. If an exercise or activity produces pain, shortness of breath, or excessive tiredness, stop doing it and seek your doctor's advice if necessary. Physical exercise that is too vigorous can actually increase cortisol. Here are some other guidelines and precautions for prenatal exercise to keep in mind:

- If you haven't been following an exercise program already, start slowly.
- Maintain a comfortably correct posture. Don't try to put your body into uncomfortable or contorted positions.
- You should be able to walk and talk comfortably while exercising without feeling or sounding breathless.
- As a general rule, exercise three to five times per week for up to 30 minutes each day.
- Avoid rigorous bouncing and arching your back.

- Do not bring your feet over your hips (for example, by assuming the bicycling-in-the-air position). Do not do sit-ups where you bend more than 45 degrees.
- Breathe continually while exercising; do not hold your breath. Normally, exhale on exertion.
- Drink a lot of fluids before, during, and after exercising to prevent dehydration.

As you progress in your pregnancy, your exercise program will change. For example, a routine that was easy for you to do early on may become too taxing in your last trimester. Consult your physician about the best amount of exercise for you, as each person is different. Any exercise program or video you choose should follow the American College of Obstetricians and Gynecologists (ACOG) guidelines. You can find those guidelines at the following websites:

http://www.acog.org/Education_and_Events
  (then visit the bookstore for several choices)

http://sales.acog.org/bookstore/_P553.cfm

Physical Resources

Prenatal Exercises	+2 pts/10 mins	🌀🌀
Prenatal Yoga	+3 pts/10 mins	🌀🌀🌀
Laughter Yoga	+20 pts/10 mins	🌀🌀🌀🌀🌀
Chiropractic Adjustment	+10 pts/adjustment	🌀🌀🌀
Enjoy Nature	+5 pts/30 mins	🌀🌀🌀
Exercise Routine	+2 pts/15 mins	🌀🌀

Prenatal Exercises

Relaxation Credit Value: +2 points for each 10 minutes of exercise

Overview

Prenatal exercises are activities designed to focus your mind in a healthy direction to help dissolve accumulated stress. Much of the stress you feel during pregnancy is due to the physiological changes your body experiences. The benefits of regular exercise during pregnancy include relieving back pain and improving posture. Your increased flexibility and strengthened muscles will help to support labor and promote feelings of well-being while reducing fatigue.

Description

The following basic prenatal exercises are for increasing your strength and flexibility and reducing your stress.

Exercise #1: Arm/upper back stretch (5 repetitions)

Step 1: Raise your arms over your head. Keep your elbows straight and the palms of your hands facing one another. Hold for at least 20 seconds.

Step 2: Lower your arms down to your side. Keep your upper back straight.

Step 3: Move your arms toward your back and stretch.

Exercise #2: Pelvic tilt (5 repetitions)

Step 1: The pelvic tilt can be done in several positions: lying on your back with your knees bent, sitting or standing up, or on your hands and knees.

Step 2: Inhale through your nose and gently tighten your stomach and buttock muscles.

Step 3: Flatten the small of your back and allow your pelvis to gently tilt upward. Hold for a count of five as you exhale slowly.

Exercise #3: Modified sit-ups (5 repetitions)

Step 1: Lie on your back with your knees bent, arms at your sides. Slowly breathe in through your nose.

Step 2: Blow out your air as you raise your head, tuck your chin gently, and lift your shoulders off the floor (less than 45 degrees).

Other Ways to Use

1. You can follow one or more of the basic exercises with a short walk or dance to some music, work out on the elliptical machine, or do some other light aerobic activity.

2. The following sit-up variations will strengthen various parts of your abdomen, depending on where you place your hands and arms. Do sit-ups at each of the following positions one to three times each at first and work up to more repetitions when you feel you are able to do so comfortably.

   • Place both of your hands on your forehead and then, as you blow out your breath, raise your head, tuck in your chin gently, and lift your shoulders slightly off the mat.

   • Cross your arms over your chest and do the sit-up.

   • Place both of your hands under your ribs and do the sit-up.

   • Place your hands on your belly button and do the sit-up.

   • Place your hands on your pelvis and do the sit-up.

Where to Find and Costs

Prenatal exercises do not cost anything to do. You can find pregnancy exercise DVDs that you can purchase and follow along with by searching the web. An excellent summary of information on exercise during pregnancy can be found at the BeFitMom website:

http://www.befitmom.com/aerobic_exercise.html

The Breech Tilt exercise that may help prevent breech positioning prior to delivery can be found here:

http://spinningbabies.com/techniques/242-breech-tilt

Resource Guide Rating

Prenatal Yoga

Relaxation Credit Value: +3 points for each 10 minutes of yoga

Overview

Yoga can be beneficial in reducing anxiety and developing peace of mind. Practicing prenatal yoga can help prevent stretch marks, excess weight gain, and back pain. Yoga can also help you to build the core strength and flexibility that you'll need to respond to the demands of childbirth and childcare.

Yoga classes that offer pregnancy groups are usually available in larger cities. If a live class is not available where you live, DVDs that specifically address all phases of pregnancy can be found by searching the Internet. If you have never participated in a class or worked out with a DVD before, remember that the person who is leading the class has been doing those poses and exercises *much* longer than you have. Do not add to your stress by trying to do what they do in exactly the way they are doing it. A rule of thumb is to do the routines at about 25 to 35 percent effort three to five times. If you are not sore afterward, you can add a little bit more effort as long as you feel good after your class and have no pain.

Description

Some of the yoga poses that are considered to be good for pregnancy include Cat-Cow, Warrior II, Triangle Pose, Pigeon Pose, Fire Log Pose, Half Moon Pose, Cobbler's Pose, Seated Forward Bend, and Side Angle Pose. If you do not already practice yoga, the best way to learn is to take a class with a good instructor who is experienced in prenatal classes. If that is not possible for you, following a DVD is another option.

Other Ways to Use

Do your yoga outside in a park or beautiful space on a pretty day.

Where to Find and Costs

Finding certified or properly qualified yoga instructors or classes in your area may be as easy as checking the phone book, talking to other mothers and friends, or searching the Internet. If you want to purchase one of the many prenatal yoga DVDs on the market, go to a bookstore or the Internet to search for the best option for you.

Resource Guide Rating

Laughter Yoga

Relaxation Credit Value: +20 points for
each 10 minutes of laughing

Overview

Laughter is one of the best stress-reduction tools available. Laughter reduces pain, increases job performance, connects people emotionally, and improves the flow of oxygen to the heart and brain.[2] Laughter Yoga, developed in 1995 by a physician in India, is revolutionary, easy to do, and produces profound physiological and psychological benefits. Laughter Yoga combines laughter with yogic breathing (pranayama). It's a fun and engaging mental activity that clears the mind and lightens the heart. Laughter Yoga is based on a scientific fact that the body cannot differentiate between forced and real laughter. Laughter Yoga is usually practiced as a group exercise where the members begin by generating "unconditional" laughter (without jokes or comedy). It soon turns into real and contagious laughter.

People who practice Laughter Yoga report significant general health improvements. A Laughter Yoga session results in positive energy that makes it easy to cope with the stress of daily life. The impact of laughter is so profound that some practitioners claim that they no longer need antidepressants. Many have experienced a reduction in the frequency of respiratory infections like the common cold and flu. In fact, an article published in August 2010 in *New Yorker Magazine* reported that Dr. Andrew Weil said that laughter yoga could lower American health-care costs.

Description

The best way to see how Laughter Yoga works is to watch a video on the website listed below.

Other Ways to Use

Laughter Yoga is a stress-reduction technique that is so life-changing that you do not need other ways to use it.

Where to Find and Costs

There are Laughter Yoga Clubs around the world. Volunteers trained as Laughter Yoga Teachers and Laughter Yoga Leaders run these social clubs. Participation in the clubs is usually free or they can be joined for only a minimal cost. For a list of available clubs worldwide, visit one of these main websites:

http://www.laughteryoga.org

http://www.laughteryogaamerica.com/

Resource Guide Rating

Chiropractic for Expectant Moms

Relaxation Credit Value: +10 points for each adjustment visit

Overview

Chiropractic care can be a great way to eliminate and manage the physical aches and pains that some expecting mothers experience. As a chiropractic adjustment relaxes tense and painful regions of the body, endorphins (a hormone that provides the body with a sense of well-being) can be released.

Pain can be a large source of stress during pregnancy, interrupting sleep and relaxation patterns. Chiropractic care for pregnant moms releases irritation, pinched nerves, and restricted mobility naturally without medication. If you suffered with lower back and neck problems or headaches before becoming pregnant, the changes of your body's structure to accommodate your growing baby will put extra stress on those areas and most likely will cause you pain while pregnant.

When pregnant, lower back pain commonly occurs as the weight of the baby shifts your center of gravity. This shift stresses the alignment of your pelvis and the stability of your lower back. As the baby grows, you have to stretch the rest of your back more to physically reach places you could easily reach before. The most common complaint during pregnancy is back pain, sciatica, and hip pain.

Description

Not only is chiropractic treatment safe for the expecting mother, it is highly recommended. There are over a dozen chiropractic techniques to treat your spine gently and precisely without force or injury. While the standard manual adjustment is easily adapted for the pregnant mother, other popular techniques that you can read more about on the web are acti-vator methods, upper cervical technique, bioelectric synchro-nization technique (B.E.S.T.), and sacral occipital technique (SOT).

Other Ways to Use

1. In addition to helping relieve back pain and discomfort during your pregnancy, chiropractors can provide support for proper alignment of the baby in the womb, help you and your baby recover from the physical stress of delivery, and help your baby adjust to the new demands of living outside the womb.

2. Chiropractic care for the newborn has been found to be extremely helpful for colic and hiccups.

3. Chiropractic care can also help women become pregnant.

Where to Find and Costs

The best place to find a good chiropractic physician is by word of mouth. Cost for chiropractic treatments can range from $55 to $135 per treatment. Many medical insurance plans offer chiropractic benefits, so be sure to check with your provider. Visit these websites for more information:

http://www.ivillage.com/chiropractic-can-chiropractic -care-help-during-pregnancy/6-a-144743

http://www.activator.com/

Resource Guide Rating

Enjoy Nature

Relaxation Credit Value: +5 points for each 30 minutes of exercise

Overview

For many of us, being out in the beauty of nature provides peace of mind. Nature, Mother Earth, can take away your stress and troubles. Sitting or strolling as you enjoy the sounds of the wind in the trees, a babbling brook, or the songs of the birds can soothe the mind and feed the soul. Allow yourself to be entertained and rejuvenated as you watch a drama between bird and squirrel unfold at the bird feeder or watch adult cardinals teaching their babies to fly. Hummingbirds and butterflies feeding on the flowers can bring a peaceful joy. Sit or walk as it starts to sprinkle and smell the earth as it absorbs the newly fallen rain.

Description

Early morning or evenings are the best times to be out in nature for a walk or simply to relax and enjoy your surroundings. The lighting is more filtered and there is a special radiance at those times of day. Stay safe and dress appropriately to avoid insect bites.

Other Ways to Use

1. The sounds of nature can often be drowned out by the noise of cars in a city or neighborhood. If that is the case where you live, take your iPod or smart phone with you and listen to a recording of nature sounds or relaxing music.

2. Sit quietly for a few minutes and incorporate breathing exercises or meditation, feed the ducks, or add other ways to help you enjoy the moment.

Where to Find and Costs

Unless you choose a park with a fee, there is no expense.

Resource Guide Rating

Exercise Routine

Relaxation Credit Value: +2 points for each 15 minutes
of exercise (to a maximum of 4 points)

Overview

Many women have an exercise routine before they become
pregnant. The guidelines and precautions for continuing your
exercise routine after you become pregnant can be found
at several places on the web, but none are more authoritative than those from the American College of Obstetricians
and Gynecologists (ACOG), described at the beginning of
the Physical Resources section (pages 226 to 227). There are
many benefits from a good exercise program, such as controlling excessive weight gain, reducing swelling of your legs and
hands, and improving posture and circulation.

Description

The ACOG recommends that pregnant women who have
been cleared for exercise by their physicians engage in approximately 30 minutes of moderate physical activity daily.
Listen to your body. Walking, swimming, moderate-intensity
aerobics, and cycling are generally safe during pregnancy.
You can continue more strenuous exercise in moderation if
you were active in sports and strength training prior to your
pregnancy.

Other Ways to Use

Take along your iPod or smart phone to listen to music while
exercising.

Where to Find and Costs

Depends on if you belong to a gym or have workout equipment in your home.

Resource Guide Rating

OVERVIEW OF
BIOFEEDBACK RESOURCES

TEMPERATURE, HEART RATE, blood pressure, and rate of breathing increase with stress and decrease with relaxation. While you can count the number of breaths you take easily enough, it is harder to be aware of blood pressure and heart-rate changes when stressed. Biofeedback uses a device or instrument to give you a signal, such as a light or beep, to help you learn to control body responses. A biofeedback device could, for example, give you a beep as your body temperature goes down and a different tone as your temperature goes up. You can use the beeps and tones as cues to help train yourself to control your body temperature. The same principle is applied to stress responses of increased heart rate and galvanic skin response. Biofeedback devices are easy to use and vary in cost.

Biofeedback Devices

StressErasure	+5 pts/10 mins	
emWave Personal Stress Reliever	+5 pts/10mins	
Stress Thermometer/Stress Card/ Mood Card	+3 pts/10 mins	
GSR2 Biofeedback Relaxation System	+5 pts/10 mins	

StressErasure

Relaxation Credit Value: +5 points for each 10-minute use

Overview

The StressErasure is an FDA approved, portable biofeedback device designed to help people respond to the habit of shallow, rapid breathing and holding their breath when really stressed. StressEraser uses a harmless infrared sensor on the fingertip that generates visual cues on a screen. This technique can help you learn to consciously change the way you breathe. The goal is to slow down your breathing to decrease the speed of your heart rate and maximize your body's natural ability to relax.

Description

The StressErasure device comes with instructions and is simple to use.

Step 1: Get into a comfortable position and take a few easy breaths. Follow directions for contact with the machine.

Step 2: Breathe in and time the moment of your exhalation for when the triangle appears on the screen.

Other Ways to Use

The StressErasure can be used when traveling. You can also play music in the background while working with it.

Where to Find and Costs

The cost ranges from approximately $100 to $200 depending on whether the equipment is new, owned before, or refurbished. Website information:

http://stresseraser.com/

Resource Guide Rating

emWave2 Personal Stress Reliever
(from HeartMath)

Relaxation Credit Value: +5 pts for each 10 minutes of use

Overview

The emWave Personal Stress Reliever is designed to reduce stress by training the user to enter a state of coherence, characterized by harmony, order, and optimal functioning in psychological (mental and emotional) as well as physiological (bodily) processes. The emWave Personal Stress Reliever is a handheld device that helps the user link their attention to the intention of generating and sustaining positive emotional feelings.

The device objectively monitors the heart's rhythms and confirms when the coherence state is achieved. With practice, it is possible to learn to shift into coherence at will, even in a difficult or super-stressful situation. This technique will be a bit more technical for some, but it does have a short learning curve. The benefit is that you will learn how to manage your stress in a proactive way.

Description

The emWave comes with a training CD and you are entitled to a free, 30-minute interactive online course to help you learn to use it efficiently. Free one-hour teleclasses are also available.

Other Ways to Use

Many applications and products using this technology are available at the HeartMath online store (see below).

Where to Find and Costs

Prices range from around $150 to $250. New and used units are available at Amazon.com and other locations. Website information:

http://www.heartmathstore.com/item/6300/emwave
-personal-stress-reliever

Resource Guide Rating

Stress Thermometer/Stress Card/Mood Card

Relaxation Credit Value: +3 points for each 10 minutes of use

Overview

Some biofeedback tools are based on the concept that when our bodies are relaxed, our hands often become warmer. When we are stressed, blood flow to our hands is reduced because of tightened muscles. Biofeedback devices that indicate stress by reduced hand temperature are readily available. The Stress Thermometer, the Stress Card (as seen on *The Dr. Oz Show*), and a Mood Card are three examples.

These items are simple, very reasonably priced biofeedback devices that measure the warmth of the hands and provide feedback using different values. The Stress Thermometer displays numbers, the Stress Card uses words, and the Mood Card works like the 70s version of the mood ring and displays colors. Hand temperatures do vary widely among people. If you notice that your normally warm hands seem to become cool and clammy when you are stressed or tense, this may be a great tool for you.

Description

The devices come with instructions for how to use.

Other Ways to Use

While you are working with one of these devices, you can add music along with gentle breathing to help you relax even more.

Where to Find and Costs

The cost varies depending on what you buy and range from approximately $10 to $30. To find out more, visit:

http://www.cliving.org/stressthermometer.htm

Resource Guide Rating

GSR2 Biofeedback Relaxation System

Relaxation Credit Value: +5 points for each 10 minutes of use

Overview

The GSR2 Biofeedback Relaxation device uses the galvanic skin response (GSR), one of the oldest of the biofeedback systems. GSR is a way of measuring tiny changes in skin pore size and in sweat gland activity at the level of the skin on your fingers, which is a relative measure of skin conductance (electrical conductance of the skin, a measure of psychological and physiological arousal of the sympathetic nervous system). As you relax, your skin conductance changes. This biofeedback device uses the changes in conductance to measure changes in your stress level. A tone is paired with the change in stress. If the tone goes up, your stress is going up. If the tone goes down, your stress is going down. The machine is small and lightweight.

Description

Step 1. Place your fingers on the device in the proper orientation.

Step 2. Try to make the tone go lower and lower (indicating that your stress is going down) as you focus on your breathing and listen to the tone in the background.

Other Ways to Use

This small device can work well if you take the time to learn how to use it. If it works for you, consider taking it with you during the day so you can check your stress levels during your daily routine. If you find that your levels are high, you can take a short break and use this device to bring yourself back to a more calm state.

Where to Find and Costs

The GSR2 Biofeedback Relaxation device costs approximately $75 and is available through many distributors. Here is one source:

http://www.toolsforwellness.com/biofeedback.html

Resource Guide Rating

OVERVIEW OF
PERSONAL PAMPERING

WITH THE MULTITUDE of demands on an expecting mom, taking a few moments of simple grooming or self-care can seem overly indulgent. If you cannot shift your focus off the tasks at hand, you might well associate the words *indulge*, *spoil*, or *coddle* with the word *pamper*. Instead, think of pampering as "treating yourself with great kindness." Practicing the art of indulging and coddling with free and healthy activities that make you feel comfortable and loved will prepare you to do the same for your baby.

With that in mind, the self-care activities included here are designed to help you show yourself that you care enough to set aside time during your day to do something "nonuseful"—something that is specifically intended to be relaxing. So when engaging in your preferred form of personal pampering, be sure to disconnect for a few minutes. Turn off the phone, lower the lights, and make this moment a little special.

Personal Pampering Ideas

Curl Up with a Good Book or Movie	+2 pts/60 mins	👓👓
Warm Bath	+3 pts/each time	👓👓
Herbal Tea Break	+5 pts/each time	👓👓
Power Nap	+10 pts/each time	👓👓👓
Sit Down and Put Up Your Feet	+2 pts/20 mins	👓👓
Sleep	+1 pt/60 mins	👓👓👓
Massage for Expecting Moms	+5 pts/30 mins	👓👓👓

Curl Up with a Good Book or Movie

Relaxation Credit Value: +2 points for each 60 minutes

Overview

For this activity of relaxing with a good book or movie, you have a vast number of choices available. There are different strokes for different folks. While reading or watching a love story or something funny may be relaxing to you at times, there may be days when you might feel better watching someone blow things up. It's all a matter of what works to reduce your stress at that point in time.

Description

Take an inventory of your mood at the moment. Think about a specific book or movie and take another inventory of your mood. Are you smiling? Do you feel a sense of relief or relaxation? If so, then that's the right choice to help you with this pampering activity.

Take a few moments to prepare yourself, creating a time and space where you will be uninterrupted, and then sit back and indulge. I used the words *curl up* in the title of this section to remind you to let your body get comfortable. Put your feet up, wrap yourself in a little blanket, rest in an easy chair or on the sofa, and enjoy your personal downtime.

Other Ways to Use

1. If it's impossible to take an hour for this activity, you can give yourself 1 point for every 30 minutes of time you take to curl up with a good book or movie.

2. Watching a two-hour movie that reduces your stress will earn you 4 points!

3. Make it a date and plan to do this with your partner.

4. Sitting on the side of the tub to soak your feet while you read a good book also qualifies as a moment of "curling up."

Where to Find and Costs

You can do this activity at home or as an outing to the library, the bookstore, the movies, or the theatre. Depending on the source of your entertainment, this activity could be free or cost just a few dollars.

Resource Guide Rating

Warm Bath

Relaxation Credit Value: +3 points for a warm bath

Overview

There is something about a bath that can be very therapeutic. Warm water is soothing, and immersion in a warm bath can release muscle tension and induce a relaxation response that provides you with a feeling of rest. Taking a bath can slow down your mind, your movement, and your words as well as deepen your sleep.

Precautions

Baths can be a potential source of infection. If you are predisposed to bladder infection, avoid using the warm bath as a relaxation technique. The American College of Obstetricians and Gynecologists recommends that a pregnant mother avoid raising her core temperature above 102 degrees at all times during pregnancy.[3] Keeping the water at 100 degrees or less is generally acceptable and most frequently recommended at all stages of pregnancy. Make sure that someone is available to help you get in and out of the tub safely if needed when you are in the later stages of pregnancy.

Description

Prepare your environment to get the most out of this pampering exercise. Warm up the bathroom enough to take the chill out of the air and lower the lights a bit if you can. Adding a light fragrance of a relaxing scent such as rose or lavender can enhance the experience.

Other Ways to Use

1. An alternative to getting into the bathtub is to simply sit on the edge of the tub and soak your feet.

2. Bring a towel into the bathtub with you, wet it, and let it rest over your tummy and breasts or your head and shoulders. That will help make your body feel a little warmer and give you the feeling of submersion.

Where to Find and Costs

As long as you have a bathtub and hot water in your house, this activity is easy to do and free.

Resource Guide Rating

Herbal Tea Break

Relaxation Credit Value: +5 points for each tea break

Overview

Relaxing with a warm cup of herbal tea can be just the thing to calm you down and help you get back in balance. There is a lot of conflicting information about the use of herbs and herbal tea during pregnancy, however. Tea companies that produce herbal tea will often list a warning on the box if a substance is known to be harmful during pregnancy. If you have doubts or questions, do your own research with the help of your medical doctor or midwife before choosing your tea. The following is the Canadian Health Authority list of approved tea for use during pregnancy: lemon balm, rose hips, orange peel, citrus peel, and ginger. A lightly flavored hot cup of tea without caffeine is a soothing and relaxing beverage. You can make a lightly flavored cup of tea by passing the tea bag through the water or allowing it to rest within a teapot for less than three minutes.

Description

The art of brewing tea is a ritual in many countries. Here are a few suggestions: The cup you use to drink your tea should make you feel special. The water should be hot but not boiling. Sit or stand quietly, wrap your hands around that warm cup, and sip. Close your eyes for a moment and relax.

Other Ways to Use

It's well known that a cup of hot water (without any tea added) can assist the bowels to move. Try adding a squeeze of lemon, lime, grapefruit, pineapple, or ginger.

Where to Find and Costs

You can easily find tea that is appropriate to drink during pregnancy. You can also make your tea with anything that you feel inclined to use to flavor a cup of hot water.

Resource Guide Rating

Power Nap

Relaxation Credit Value: +10 pts for a power nap

Overview

Viewpoints on the definition of a power nap vary widely. I see it as a short rest that provides the benefits of having rested for a longer amount of time and meets these four criteria:

- It lasts less than 45 minutes.

- You've achieved and sustained total relaxation for a few minutes during that time.

- You wake up without an alarm when you have had enough rest (usually about 15 minutes).

- You arise refreshed and renewed as if you have been asleep for an hour or more.

My own personal power nap lasts 7 to 8 minutes. I hear myself breathing deeply, I feel as if I am drifting . . . drifting . . . drifting, and I am gone. I wake up feeling more rested. A friend of mine, whose power naps last 18 minutes, describes a power nap as "the achievement of total relaxation, where you feel as if you could not move your body at all, even if you tried."

Description

Step 1: Take your shoes off. Lie down and put your head on a pillow or recline in a chair with a little cover over you.

Step 2: Rest. Slow down your breathing.

Step 3: Begin to feel heavier and heavier until you cannot move, even if you tried to. Stay that way until you feel that that is enough time for you. Rouse yourself from your rest state and look at the clock. Did more than

15 minutes and less than 45 minutes pass? You have just experienced a power nap.

Other Ways to Use

Designate 15 minutes a day for a power nap if you can. Schedule it at lunchtime, when you come home from work, or after doing other activities. If you make this a habit, your body will grow accustomed to taking a power nap, and it will become easier and easier for you to enter this state of relaxation quickly.

Where to Find and Costs

A power nap doesn't cost anything but your time.

Resource Guide Rating

👓 👓 👓

Sit Down and Put Up Your Feet

Relaxation Credit Value: +2 pts for every 20 minutes

Overview

There is something powerful about simply putting your feet up. It speaks the word *relaxation* to your body. If you do this often enough, your body will begin to listen and respond with relaxation whenever you do this. The only additional thing you need for this activity is to intentionally shift your focus to doing something peaceful.

Description

Sit down where it is quiet and comfortable for you. Put your feet up on something and take a break from your normal routine. You can also lie in a comfortable position on the floor, making sure to support your back and head, and put your feet up.

Other Ways to Use:

1. Add some music.

2. Add a smile or some laughs.

3. Play a little mindless game.

4. Catch up on a friendly phone call.

Where to Find and Costs

An easy way to put your feet up is to sit in a reclining chair if you have one. If you want to lie on the floor to relax, you can put your feet up onto a sofa or any chair. A pillow, a towel, or even a coat used as a pillow can soften up any surface.

Resource Guide Rating

Sleep

Relaxation Credit Value: +1 pt for
each hour of restful sleep

Overview

A woman requires extra nutrition and extra rest while pregnant. The body needs time to erase the stress of the day.
Restful sleep is not as easy as it sounds when your sleeping
positions are altered by the needs of the baby and the cautions of your attending physician. In addition, the baby's body
movements and position can frequently awaken you to go to
the bathroom during the night. Your thoughts, schedule, and
concern about the never-ending to-do list can also delay or
interrupt your sleep cycle. So when you get extra sleep, you
get extra credit.

Description

Sleep is the one pleasure that needs no description.

Other Ways to Use

You can also give yourself one additional point of credit for
each half hour before normal bedtime that you go to bed.

Where to Find and Costs

The only cost of giving yourself more time to sleep is taking
something else off your daily schedule, knowing that the benefits of more sleep while you are pregnant—to yourself and
your baby—are huge.

Resource Guide Rating

Massage for Expecting Moms

Relaxation Credit Value: +5 points for
each 30 minutes of massage

Overview

Massage can reduce stress and anxiety when you are pregnant, and massage therapists can be instrumental in improving your comfort. Massage can also induce deep relaxation and a restful state as well as improve your body's ability to restore and reenergize. While chiropractors can help your body's structure adapt to being pregnant, massage therapists can help your body's tissues adapt to the changes that occur in pregnancy.

Description

Many styles of massage are helpful to the expecting mom. You can receive a massage while you are lying on your side and while you are supported with pillows made especially for massaging pregnant women. To learn more about prenatal massage, visit:

http://www.americanpregnancy.org/pregnancyhealth/
prenatalmassage.html

Other Ways to Use

Most massage therapists play relaxing music during their work and sometimes you can bring along a CD that you want to hear while receiving the massage.

Where to Find and Costs

Ask friends for referrals or call massage therapists yourself to ask if they have experience working with expecting mothers.

You can also find a list of massage therapists in your area who are specially trained and registered with the American Pregnancy Organization here:

http://www.americanpregnancy.org/members/
massagetherapists

Resource Guide Rating

Notes

Chapter 1: An Ounce of Prevention

1. For information on the changes that happen in your body during pregnancy, consult your physician first as well as several excellent resources like Heidi Murkoff's book *What to Expect When You're Expecting;* the Internet site www.pregnancyguide online.com; *The Working Woman's Pregnancy Book* by Marjorie Greenfield; and Annie Murphy Paul's new bestseller, *Origins: How the Nine Months Before Birth Shape the Rest of Our Lives.*

2. Margaret R. Oates, "Adverse effects of maternal antenatal anxiety on children: causal effect or developmental continuum?" *British Journal of Psychiatry 180* (2002): 478–79.

   Dr. Oates is a psychiatrist in Britain who opined in this article that it is dangerous to alert the public to dangers without possible treatments. As I noted in chapter 1, however, I believe that women should know about and understand the research on prenatal stress that has been conducted so far. We know enough about the potential risks of unreduced prenatal stress that it's wise for women to learn how to use stress-reduction techniques consistently while pregnant.

Chapter 2: Today's Pregnant Mom Has More to Manage

1. Calvin J. Hobel et al., "Maternal plasma corticotropin-releasing hormone associated with stress at 20 weeks' gestation in pregnancies ending in preterm delivery," *American Journal of Obstetrics and Gynecology 180* (1999): S257–63. Dr. Hobel and his team have published many important papers describing how stress increases the risk for preterm birth. This particular article explains one of his primary findings.

   Vivette Glover, "Annual Research Review: Prenatal stress

and the origins of psychopathology: an evolutionary perspective," *Journal of Child Psychology and Psychiatry* 52 (2011): 356–67. Dr. Glover's review on prenatal stress and psychopathology is excellent and reviews the major work published up to 2011. Dr. Glover is also a key member of the research team at Avon, England, with the Children of the 90s project. The Avon project is described in more detail in chapter 6.

Chapter 3: What Busy Schedules and Busy Minds Do to Us

1. Cortisol is released by the adrenal cortex, small organs on top of the kidney, in response to the pituitary gland in the brain sending a message to the adrenal gland. The message originates at the hypothalamus in the brain. Thus, this chain reaction is called the HPA (hypothalamus-pituitary-adrenal) axis.

2. Keith J. Karren et al., *Mind/Body Health: The Effects of Attitudes, Emotions, and Relationships*, 4th ed. (San Francisco: Benjamin Cummings, 2009). Metabolic syndrome is a group of risk factors, including high insulin resistance, high blood pressure, and excessive fat around the waist.

3. Hans Selye, "Stress and disease," *Science* 122 (1955): 625–31. Dr. Hans Selye was a Hungarian-born, pioneering endocrinologist who was the first person to coin the term *stress*. In 1950 Dr. Selye published a thousand-page opus on the science, theory, and medical implications of stress called *The Physiology and Pathology of Exposure to Stress*.

4. The following two studies are a sample of information that has been published on the physical, mental, and emotional effects of long-term exposure to stress by adults: Sonja J. Lupien et al., "Cortisol levels during human aging predict hippocampal atrophy and memory deficits," *Nature Neuroscience* 1 (1998): 69–73; Letizia Bossini et al., "Magnetic resonance imaging volumes of the hippocampus in drug-naïve patients with post-traumatic stress disorder without comorbidity conditions," *Journal of Psychiatric Research* 42 (2008): 752–62.

5. The hippocampus is in the brain. It stores our long-term memories and helps us with visual-spatial types of tasks, such as finding our way around our environment, making a mental

map of where we have been, or other important things such as reading the time on a clock.

Chapter 4: The Alarming Rise in Childhood Disorders

1. Joseph Chilton Pearce, *The Magical Child* (New York: Plume Books, 1977), 28.
2. Attention deficit disorders include attention deficit disorder and attention deficit hyperactivity disorder. They are defined in the *Diagnostic and Statistical Manual for Mental Disorder-IV-TR* (Washington, D. C.: American Psychiatric Association, 1994).
3. Graham J. Emslie, "Pediatric Anxiety—Underrecognized and Undertreated," *New England Journal of Medicine* 359 (2008): 2835–36.
4. Jeffrey J. Wood et al., "Parenting and childhood anxiety: theory, empirical endings, and future directions," *Journal of Child Psychology* 44 (2003): 134–51.
5. Lauren S. Wakschlag et al., "Maternal Smoking During Pregnancy and the Risk of Conduct Disorder in Boys," *Archives General Psychiatry* 54 (1997): 670–76.

Chapter 5: The Body's Amazing Changes during Pregnancy

1. American College of Obstetricians and Gynecologists, *Your Pregnancy and Childbirth: Month to Month*, 5th ed. (Washington, D. C.: American College of Obstetrician and Gynecologists, 2010).
2. Elaine M. Scott et al., "The Increase in Plasma and Saliva Cortisol Levels in Pregnancy Is Not Due to the Increase in Corticosteroid-Binding Globulin Levels," *Journal of Clinical Endocrinology and Metabolism* 71 (1990): 639–44.

Chapter 6: Landmark Studies on Pregnancy and Stress

1. Vivette Glover, "Annual Research Review: Prenatal stress and the origins of psychopathology: an evolutionary perspective," *Journal of Child Psychology and Psychiatry* 52 (2011): 356–67.
2. The following articles are a good sample of the seminal animal

studies on prenatal stress: William R. Thompson, "Influence of prenatal maternal anxiety on emotionality in young rats," *Science* 125 (1957): 698–99; Mary L. Schneider and Christopher L. Coe, "Repeated social stress during pregnancy impairs neuromotor development of the primate infant," *Journal of Developmental and Behavioral Pediatrics* 14 (1993): 81–87; Mary L Scheider, Colleen F. Moore, Gary W. Kraemer, Andrew D. Roberts, and Onofre T. DeJesus, "The impact of prenatal stress, fetal alcohol exposure, or both on development: perspectives from a primate model," *Psychoneuroendocrinology* 27 (2002): 285–98; Anja C Huizink, Eduard J. H. Mulder, Pascale G. Robles de Medina, Gerard H. A. Visser, and Jan K. Buitelaar, "Is pregnancy anxiety a distinctive syndrome?" *Early Human Development* 79 (2004): 81–91.

3. Jim van Os and Jean-Paul Selten, "Prenatal exposure to maternal stress and subsequent schizophrenia. The May 1940 invasion of The Netherlands," *British Journal of Psychiatry* 172 (1998): 324–26.

4. David P. Laplante, Alain Brunet, Norbert Schmitz, Antonio Ciampi, and Suzanne King, "Project Ice Storm: prenatal maternal stress affects cognitive and linguistic functioning in 5½ year-old children," *Journal of the American Academy of Child and Adolescent Psychiatry* 47 (2008): 1063–72.

This study involves 89 children of mothers who were pregnant during the January 1998 ice storm in Quebec. The mothers were placed into three groups (mild, moderate, and high stress during the storm) on the basis of both objective and subjective measures. The children were assessed at age 5½ years using three subtests of the Wechsler Preschool and Primary Scales of Intelligence-Revised (Similarities, Information, and Block Design) and the Peabody Picture Vocabulary Test-Revised. Block Design was not negatively affected.

There are several important findings from this study: (1) Children of mothers who experienced high stress during the severe ice storm scored significantly lower on Full Scale IQ and on scales that measure verbal abstract reasoning and information as compared to children of mothers who experienced moderate or low stress during the same natural disaster. (2) The study suggests that timing of the exposure to the natural disaster is important, with poorer outcomes associated with first and second trimester exposure. (3) The negative effects associated with prenatal stress were seen at 2 years, 5 ½ years, and 8 ½ years of age, indicating relatively long-lasting effects. (4) There is an ongoing MRI study to determine if the observed differences in intellectual, behavioral, and emotional development between children of mothers who experienced greater versus lower amounts of stress could be mediated by differences in brain development.

5. The Avon Longitudinal Study of Parents and Children (ALSPAC) was originally called the Avon Longitudinal Study of Pregnancy and Childhood and is also known as the Avon study or the Children of the 90s study.

6. For more information on the Children of the 90s ongoing research, publications, and press releases, visit http://www. alspac.bristol.ac.uk/.

7. Simon de Bruxelles, "How Harriet Is Changing the World for Children," *The Times*, October 23, 2004.

8. Thomas G. O'Connor, Jonathan Heron, Jean Golding, Michael Beveridge, and Vivette Glover, "Maternal antenatal anxiety and children's behavioural/emotional problems at 4 years. Report from the Avon Longitudinal Study of Parents and Children," *British Journal of Psychiatry* 180 (2002): 502–8; Thomas G. O'Connor, Jonathan Heron, Vivette Glover, and the ALSPAC Study Team, "Antenatal anxiety predicts child behavioral/emotional problems independently of postnatal depression," *Journal of the American Academy of Child and Adolescent Psychiatry* 41 (2002): 1470–77.

9. The entire sample from the Avon study includes approximately 14,000 mother-child pairs. The 2002 published articles reported on a smaller sample of 7,448 for several reasons. The data were collected over several assessment times. To be in these particular data analyses, all questionnaires from all time points needed to have been collected within a specified time frame. That caused a drop in the total number of mother-child

pairs included in the analyses.

10. John Birtchnell, C. Evans, and J. Kennard, "The total score of the Crown-Crisp Experiential Index: A useful and valid measure of psychoneurotic pathology," *British Journal of Medical Psychology* 61 (1988): 255–66. The Crown-Crisp Index of Phobic Anxiety measures a type of stress called phobic anxiety or self-reported fears and phobias.

11. James Elander and Michael Rutter, "Use and development of the Rutter parents' and teachers' scale," *International Journal of Methods of Psychiatric Research* 6 (1996): 63–78. The Rutter scales were used to rate the Avon children's behavior, emotional adjustment, and attention when they reached age 4.

12. O'Connor et al. reported in the 2002 article that higher levels of stress at the 32-week point of gestation were related to the greatest risk for boys (more boys than girls) to develop problems with inattention and hyperactivity. However, the risk for girls and boys were close to the same for conduct problems and emotional problems when the mothers' anxiety levels at both 18 and 32 weeks gestation were included in the analyses.

13. The percentage of women who experienced elevated anxiety (based on scoring in the top 15 percent on the Crown-Crisp Index) when their children were at either 18 weeks or 32 weeks gestational age was about 30 percent of the total, or 2,200 pregnant women. Approximately 5 percent (or 375) of the pregnant women in the Avon study reported that they were experiencing significantly elevated anxiety almost all the time they were pregnant.

O'Connor and his team reported that the number of dropouts was highest in those women with high anxiety scores at the 18-week assessment. The highest anxiety mother-child pairs were not included in the 32-week data analysis, as they had already dropped out of the study. So researchers felt that the results of the study may have *even underestimated* the effects of chronic stress and anxiety on the developing baby. The rationale for that is that because some women with the highest anxiety scores dropped out, the moms with the highest levels of stress/anxiety were not even in the final data analysis.

14. Thomas G. O'Connor, Jonathan Heron, Jean Golding, Vivette Glover, and the ALSPAC Study Team, "Maternal antenatal anxiety and behavioural/emotional problems in children: a test of a programming hypothesis," *Journal of Child Psychology and Psychiatry* 44 (2003): 1025–36.

Children whose mothers reported high levels of anxiety in late pregnancy exhibited higher rates of behavioral and emotional problems at 81 months of age. The reported problems were consistent with those reported at age 47 months. At 81 months of age (6+ years) the problems are still present.

15. Thomas. G O'Connor, Yoav Ben-Shlomo, Jonathan Heron, Jean Golding, Diana Adams, and Vivette Glover, "Prenatal Anxiety Predicts Individual Differences in Cortisol in Pre-Adolescent Children," *Biological Psychiatry* 58 (2005): 211–17.

A subsample of 74 of the Avon children at age 10 years old were asked to collect samples of saliva first thing in the morning and at three other times during the day. The samples were collected for three days. Dr. Thomas O'Connor and the study team examined the children's levels of cortisol and found that the mothers' levels of prenatal anxiety, some 10 years earlier, predicted the children's higher morning and afternoon cortisol levels. In other words, the higher the mother's cortisol levels *when she was pregnant*, the higher the child's cortisol levels 10 years later. This study is cited as providing evidence that prenatal anxiety might have lasting effects on the HPA axis functioning in the child and that the child's HPA axis is affected by the mother's high cortisol levels during pregnancy.

16. Nick Kerswell, "Mum's Anxiety Affects Unborn Baby's Brain," press release, August 31, 2001, University of Bristol, Avon Longitudinal Study of Parents and Children, http://www.bristol.ac.uk/alspac/documents/mums-anxiety.pdf.

17. Annie M. Paul, *Origins: How the Nine Months Before Birth Shape the Rest of Our Lives* (New York: Free Press, 2010).

18. Janet A. DiPietro, Sterling C. Hilton, Melissa Hawkins, Kathleen Costigan, and Eva K. Pressman, "Maternal stress and affect influence fetal neurobehavioral development," *Developmental Psychology*. 38 (2002): 659–68.

In her studies, Dr. DiPietro usually defines stress in a different way than the Avon studies do. For example, in the study cited above Dr. DiPietro et al. investigated 52 mother-child pairs at 24, 30, and 36 weeks gestation. Measures of the unborn child's behavior included fetal heart rate, variability, and motor activity. The researchers found that women who appraised their lives as more stressful and who reported more frequent pregnancy-specific hassles had babies who were more active in the womb. Women who judged their pregnancy as uplifting and who had a positive emotional feeling toward pregnancy had babies who were less active. However, as you've seen, the Avon studies reviewed in chapter 6 define and measure prenatal stress as severe anxiety or high levels of persistent stress; and the Avon studies did find a correlation between that kind of prenatal stress and a child developing problems with attention, conduct, and emotional difficulties.

Chapter 7: Childhood Problems Related to Prenatal Stress

1. Jack P. Shonkoff; Andrew S. Garner; and the Committee on Psychosocial Aspects of Child and Family Health; Committee on Early Childhood, Adoptions, and Dependent Care; and Section on Developmental and Behavioral Pediatrics, "The Lifelong Effects of Early Childhood Adversity and Toxic Stress," *Pediatrics* 129 (2012): e232–46.
2. Bea Van den Bergh and Alfons Marcoen, "High Antenatal Maternal Anxiety Is Related to ADHD Symptoms, Externalizing Problems, and Anxiety in 8- and 9-year-olds," *Child Development* 75 (2004): 1085–97.

   Van den Bergh and Marcoen's study involved 71 women and their firstborn children. First, ratings were made of the mothers' anxiety and stress levels at postmenstrual weeks 12 to 22 and at 32 to 40. Then the mother, the child, the child's teacher, and an external observer completed rating scales and measurements when the children were 8 and 9 years old. Each mother-and-child pair rated their own behavior and emotional states using, among other measures, a well-known measure called the State-Trait Anxiety Inventory. The teacher and the outside observer rated the mother's anxiety and the child's behavior when the children were school age.

3. Barbara M. Gutteling, Carolina de Weerth, and Jan K. Buitelaar, "Prenatal stress and children's cortisol reaction to the first day of school," *Psychoneuroendocrinology* 30 (2005): 541–49.

  Dr. Gutteling and her colleagues examined whether prenatal stress predicted HPA-axis reactions of children on the first day of school after the summer break. Included in the study were 29 mother-child pairs. The children were evaluated when they reached 5 years of age. The mother-child pairs were divided into two groups, mothers with more prenatal stress were compared to mothers with less prenatal stress. Both prenatal cortisol and pregnancy anxiety were related to the children's salivary cortisol levels as a reaction to the first day of school. In other words, the higher the mother's fears and cortisol levels during her pregnancy, the higher the child's cortisol levels in the new situation of the first day of school.

4. Dennis K. Kinney, Kerim M. Munir, David J. Crowley, and Andrea M. Miller, "Prenatal Stress and Risk for Autism," *Neuroscience and Biobehavioral Reviews* 32 (2008): 1519–32.

  Dr. Kinney and his colleagues provide an excellent and up-to-date review of studies relating prenatal stress and autism. One retrospective study reviewed in this article looked at prenatal records of 58 mothers of autistic children and compared the findings to records of a matched group of 59 healthy children. This study found that the mothers of the autistic children reported significantly more family discord during their pregnancy than the mothers of the matched group of healthy children.

5. An example of one of the recent studies that talks about the effects of high levels of prenatal stress on a child's IQ is David P. Laplante, Alain Brunet, Norbert Schmitz, Antonio Ciampi, and Suzanne King, "Project Ice Storm: prenatal maternal stress affects cognitive and linguistic functioning in 5½-year-old children," *Journal of the American Academy of Child and Adolescent Psychiatry* 47 (2008): 1063–72. This study is

described in note 4 for chapter 6 above.

6. Calvin J. Hobel, Christine Dunkel-Schetter, Scott C. Roesch, Lony C. Castro, and Chander P. Arora, "Maternal plasma corticotropin-releasing hormone associated with stress at 20 weeks' gestation in pregnancies ending in preterm delivery," *American Journal of Obstetrics and Gynecology* 180 (1999): S257–63; Calvin J. Hobel, A. Goldstein, and Emily S. Barrett, "Psychosocial stress and pregnancy outcome," *Clinical Obstetrics and Gynecology* 51 (2008): 333–48.

Dr. Hobel tested the hypothesis that prenatal stress is associated with elevated levels of corticotropin-releasing hormone and the activation of the placental-adrenal axis, which leads to preterm birth. Researchers assessed 524 women for stress (using the Perceived Stress Scale), anxiety (using the State Trait Inventory), and medical conditions (including hormonal assays) at three points during the pregnancy (18-20 weeks, 28-30 weeks, and 35-36 weeks). Preterm births were associated with elevated levels of CRH (corticotropin-releasing hormone) at 18-20 weeks.

7. Rosalind J. Wright, Cynthia M. Visness, Agustin Calatroni et al., "Prenatal Maternal Stress and Cord Blood Innate and Adaptive Cytokine Responses in an Inner-City Cohort," *American Journal of Respiratory and Critical Care Medicine* 182 (2010): 25-33.

The study included 557 urban, minority, low-income families from Boston, Baltimore, New York, and St. Louis. Factors of stress included financial hardships, neighborhood and domestic violence, and housing conditions. A sample of blood from the baby's umbilical cord was tested for reactions to various allergens.

8. Hannah Cookson, Raquel Granell, Carol Joinson, Yoav Ben-Shlomo, and A. John Henderson, "Mothers' anxiety during pregnancy is associated with asthma in their children," *Journal of Allergy and Clinical Immunology* 123 (2009): 847–53.

Some of the children in the Avon study were selected as they reached 7½ to 8 years old to examine the relationship of excess prenatal stress to allergies. A significant number of the children had already been to see a physician in order to be evaluated for or diagnosed with asthma and/or allergies.

Chapter 8: The Dynamics of Prenatal Stress in the Womb

1. Vivette Glover, "Annual Research Review: Prenatal stress and the origins of psychopathology: an evolutionary perspective," *Journal of Child Psychology and Psychiatry*, 52 (2011): 356–67.
2. Arnaud Charil, David P. Laplante, Cathy Vaillancourt, and Suzanne King, "Prenatal stress and brain development," *Brain Research Reviews* 65 (2010): 56–79.

    The Charil et al. paper provides a good review of animal research on prenatal stress and brain development. They review the three proposed mechanisms by which prenatal stress affects the fetus. The brain areas affected include the hippocampus, amygdala, corpus callosum and anterior commissure, cerebral cortex, cerebellum and hypothalamus. Finally, Charil et al. propose projects like their Project Ice Storm and the MRI study as a way to look at the brains of the children to determine if the same areas are affected in humans as in animals.
3. Jeronima M. Teixeira, Nicholas M. Fisk, and Vivette Glover, "Association between maternal anxiety in pregnancy and increased uterine artery resistance index: cohort based study," *British Medical Journal* 318 (1999): 153–57.

    The 100 pregnant women who participated in this study were asked to rate their stress levels using the State-Trait Anxiety measure. The researchers carried out ultrasound scans to test the blood flow through their arteries. The researchers took a "resistance index" measurement of the extent to which the blood flow was impaired and found that 27 percent of the women in the most anxious group had a resistance index high enough to potentially cause reduced fetal development and birth weight. By contrast, only 4 percent in the less anxious group had similarly impaired uterine artery blood flow.
4. Jean-Pierre Relier, "Influence of maternal stress on fetal behavior and brain development," *Biology of the Neonate* 79 (2001): 168–71.

    Dr. Relier concluded that chronic anxiety causes increased

stillbirth rate, fetal growth retardation, and altered placental morphology. He also indicated that studies have demonstrated a relationship between maternal psychological stress and increased of asphyxiation in utero.

5. Catherine Monk, Richard P. Sloan, Michael Myers, Lauren M. Ellman, Elizabeth Werner, Jiyeon Jeon, Felice Tager, and William P. Fifer, "Fetal heart rate reactivity differs by women's psychiatric status: An early marker for developmental risk," *Journal of the American Academy of Child and Adolescent Psychiatry* 43 (2004): 283–90.

The study involved 57 third-trimester pregnant women divided into two groups on the basis of their chronic anxiety before pregnancy. The pregnant woman was experimentally stressed. The fetuses of depressed and anxious women reacted to the experimental stress with increased heart rate compared to the fetuses of healthy, low-anxiety women.

6. The task Dr. Monk used to induce "stress" in the above 2004 study is a simple neuropsychological test that is often used to measure a person's ability to pay attention while simultaneously screening out competing information. It is called the Stroop Test. It takes less than 10 minutes to administer. The Stroop Test has three parts. The "stressful" part requires the person to read the color that a word is printed in instead of what the word actually says. For example, if the word BLUE is printed in red-colored type, you would be asked to say "red" instead of "blue."

7. Sarah L Berga, Marsha D. Marcus, Tammy L. Loucks et al., "Recovery of ovarian activity in women with functional hypothalamic amenorrhea who were treated with cognitive behavior therapy," *Fertility and Sterility* 80 (2003): 976–81.

In her 2003 study, Dr. Berga compared 8 women who underwent "talk" therapy with a therapist to help them reduce tension with 8 women who did not receive that relaxation training. Her study showed that ovulation was restored in 7 of the 8 women who underwent the "talk" therapy while ovulation was restored in only 2 of 8 women who did not receive that therapy.

Chapter 9: The A, B, Cs of Stress Reduction

1. Sarah L. Berga et al., "Recovery of ovarian activity in women with functional hypothalamic amenorrhea who were treated with cognitive behavior therapy," *Fertility and Sterility* 80 (2003): 976–81.
2. Christine Dunkel-Schetter, R. Gurung, Marci Lobel, and Pathik D. Wadhwa, "Psychological, biological, and social processes in pregnancy: Using a stress framework to study birth outcomes," in A. Baum, T. Revenson, and J. Singer, eds., *Handbook of Health Psychology* (Hillsdale, NJ: Erlbaum, 2000), 495–518.
3. Rosalind J. Wright et al., "Prenatal Maternal Stress and Cord Blood Innate and Adaptive Cytokine Responses in an Inner-City Cohort," *American Journal of Respiratory and Critical Care Medicine* 182 (2010): 25–33.

Chapter 11: The Power of Sound and Music for Relaxation

1. Don Campbell and Alex Doman, *Healing at the Speed of Sound* (New York: Hudson Street Press, 2011).
2. Pierre Sollier, *Listening for Wellness: An Introduction to the Tomatis Method* (Walnut Creek, CA: Mozart Center Press, 2005).
3. A. Klopfenstein, "Die Tomatis babies," in Alfred A. Tomatis, ed., *Klangwelt Mutterleib* (Munich, Germany: Kösel-Verlag, 1994), 132–56.
4. Stéphanie Khalfa, Simone Dalla Bella, Mathieu Roy, Isabelle Peretz, and Sonia J. Lupien, "effects of relaxing music on salivary cortisol level after psychological stress," *Annals of New York Academy of Science* 999 (2003): 374–76.

Chapter 12: Creating Your Personal Stress Solutions Plan

1. As I noted in chapter 11, Dr. Stéphanie Khalfa's study showed that listening to music more quickly reduced cortisol than sitting quietly and trying to relax (see page 162).

Chapter 14: Directory of Resources

1. A special music program that includes headphones with a bone-conduction capability has a greater relaxation value. Such earphones are available for purchase at enlisten.com.
2. Hara Estroff Marano, "Laughter: The Best Medicine," *Psychology Today*, April 5, 2005.
3. See American College of Obstetricians and Gynecologists, *Your Pregnancy and Childbirth: Month to Month*, 5th ed. (Washington, D.C.: American College of Obstetricians and Gynecologists, 2010), http://www.yourpregnancyandchildbirth.com/.

References and Additional Reading

American College of Obstetricians and Gynecologists. *Your Pregnancy and Childbirth: Month to Month*, 5th ed. Washington, D.C.: American College of Obstretricians and Gynecologists, 2010.

Andrews, Susan R., Janet Blumenthal, Carol Ferguson, Dale Johnson, Alfred Kahn, Tom Lasater, Paul Malone, and Doris Wallace. "The skills of mothering: A study of the Parent-Child Development Centers." *Monographs of the Society for Research in Child Development (Serial No. 198)*. Chicago: University of Chicago Press, 1982.

Akakios, Andrianna, and Wynand F. du Plessis. "The effects of the Tomatis Method on first-time pregnant women." *Ricochet -onlinejournal.com* 2 (2009).

Benson, Hebert. *The Relaxation Response*. New York: Avon Books, 1975.

Beijers, Roseriet, Jarno Jansen, Marianne Riksen-Walraven, and Carolina de Weerth. "Maternal Prenatal Anxiety and Stress Predict Infant Illnesses and Health Complaints." *Pediatrics* 126 (2010): 401–9.

Berga, Sarah L., Marsha D. Marcus, Tammy L. Loucks, Stefanie Hlastala, Rebecca Ringham, and Marijane A. Krohn. "Recovery of ovarian activity in women with functional hypothalamic amenorrhea who were treated with cognitive behavior therapy." *Fertility and Sterility* 80 (2003): 976–81.

Birtchnell, John, C. Evans, and J. Kennard. "The total score of the Crown-Crisp Experiential Index: A useful and valid measure of psychoneurotic pathology." *British Journal of Medical Psychology* 61 (1988): 255–66.

Bossini, Letizia, Maricla Tavanti, Sara Calossi, Alessia Lombardelli, Nicola Riccardo Polizzotto, Rosita Galli, Gianpaolo Vatti,

Fulvio Pieraccini, and Paolo Castrogiovanni. "Magnetic resonance imaging volumes of the hippocampus in drug-naïve patients with post-traumatic stress disorder without comorbidity conditions." *Journal of Psychiatric Research* 42 (2008): 752–62.

Buitelaar, Jan K., Anja C. Huizink, Eduard J. H. Mulder, Pascalle G. Robles de Medina, and Gerard H. A. Visser. "Prenatal stress and cognitive development and temperament in infants." *Neurobiology of Aging* 24 (2003): S53–S60.

Buitelaar, Jan K. "Prenatal stress and risk for psychopathology early or later in life: specific effects or induction of general susceptibility?" *Psychological Bulletin* 130 (2004): 115–42.

Campbell, Don. *The Mozart Effect.* New York: Avon Books, 1997.

Campbell, Don, and Alex Doman. *Healing at the Speed of Sound: Transforming Our Lives with What We Hear.* New York: Hudson Street Press, 2011.

Chang, Meii-Yueh, Chung-Hey Chen, and Kuo-Feng Huang. "Effects of music therapy on psychological health of women during pregnancy." *Journal of Clinical Nursing* 17 (2008): 2580–87.

Charil, Arnaud, David P. Laplante, Cathy Vaillancourt, and Suzanne King. "Prenatal stress and brain development." *Brain Research Reviews* 65 (2010): 56–79.

Cookson, Hannah, Raquel Granell, Carol Joinson, Yoav Ben-Shlomo, and A. John Henderson. "Mothers' anxiety during pregnancy is associated with asthma in their children." *Journal of Allergy and Clinical Immunology* 123 (2009): 847–53.

Davis, Dorinne. *The Cycle of Sound: A Missing Link and Its Healing Implications.* Newton, New Jersey: New Pathways Press, 2012.

Dingfelder, Sadie. "Programmed for psychopathology?" *Monitor on Psychology* 35 (2004): 56.

DiPietro, Janet A., Sterling C. Hilton, Melissa Hawkins, Kathleen Costigan, and Eva K. Pressman. "Maternal stress and affect influence fetal neurobehavioral development." *Developmental Psychology* 38 (2002): 659–68.

DiPietro, Janet A., Laura E. Caulfield, Rafael A. Irizarry, Ping Chen, Mario Merialdi, and Nelly Zavaleta. "Prenatal development of intrafetal and maternal-fetal synchrony." *Behavioral Neuroscience* 120 (2006): 687–701.

Dunkel-Schetter, Christine, R. Gurung, Marci Lobel, and Pathik D. Wadhwa. "Psychological, biological, and social processes in pregnancy: Using a stress framework to study birth outcomes." In A. Baum, T. Revenson, and J. Singer, eds., *Handbook of Health Psychology*. Hillsdale, NJ: Erlbaum, 2000.

du Plessis, Wynand F., and P E. Van Jaarsveld. "Audio-psycho-phonology: A comparative outcome study on anxious primary school pupils." *South Africa Tydskr. Sielk (Journal of Psychology)* 18 (1988): 144–51.

Dyer, Wayne W. *The Power of Intention: Learning to Co-create Your World Your Way*. Carlsbad, CA: Hay House, 2005.

Elander, James, and Michael Rutter. "Use and development of the Rutter parents' and teachers' scale." *International Journal of Methods of Psychiatric Research* 6 (1996): 63–78.

Elander, James, and Michael Rutter. "An update on the status of the Rutter parents' and teachers' scales." *Child Psychology and Psychiatry Review* 1 (1996): 31–35.

Emslie, Graham J. "Pediatric Anxiety—Underrecognized and Undertreated." *New England Journal of Medicine* 359 (2008): 2835–36.

Entringer, Sonja, Robert Kumsta, Dirk H. Hellhammer, Pathik D. Wadhwa, and Stefan Wust. "Prenatal exposure to maternal psychosocial stress and HPA axis regulation in young adults." *Hormones and Behavior* 55 (2009): 292–98.

Gilmor, Tim M. "The Tomatis Method and the genesis of listening." *Pre and Peri-Natal Psychology Journal* 4 (1989): 9–26.

Gilmor, Tim M. "The efficacy of the Tomatis Method for children with learning and communication disorders: a Meta-analysis." *International Journal of Listening* 13 (1999): 12–23.

Gilmor, Tim, Paul Madaule, and Billie Thompson, eds. *About the Tomatis Method*. Toronto: Listening Centre Press, 1989.

Gladwell, Malcolm. *The Tipping Point: How Little Things Can Make a Big Difference*. New York: Back Bay Books, 2002.

Glover, Vivette. "Maternal stress or anxiety in pregnancy and emotional development of the child." *The British Journal of Psychiatry: The Journal of Mental Science* 171 (1997): 105–6.

Glover, Vivette, Thomas G. O'Connor, Jean Golding, and the ALSPAC Study Team. "Antenatal maternal anxiety is linked with atypical handedness in the child." *Early Human Development* 79 (2004): 107–18.

Glover, Vivette. "Annual Research Review: Prenatal stress and the origins of psychopathology: an evolutionary perspective." *Journal of Child Psychology and Psychiatry* 52 (2011): 356–67.

Golding, Jean. "Research Protocol: European Longitudinal Study of Pregnancy and Childhood (ELSPAC)." *Paediatric and Perinatal Epidemiology* 3 (1989): 460–69.

Golding Jean. "Children of the nineties. A longitudinal study of pregnancy and childhood based on the population of Avon (ALSPAC)." *West of England Medical Journal* 105 (1990): 80–82.

Goleman, Daniel. *Emotional Intelligence: Why It Can Matter More Than IQ.* New York: Bantam, 1995.

Greendale, Gail A., D. Kritz-Silverstein, Teresa Seeman, and Elizabeth Louise Barrett-Connor. "Higher Basal Cortisol Predicts Verbal Memory Loss in Postmenopausal Women: Rancho Bernardo Study: Brief Reports." *Journal of the American Geriatrics Society* 48 (2000): 1655–58.

Greenfield, Marjorie. *The Working Woman's Pregnancy Book.* New Haven: Yale University Press, 2008.

Gunnar, Megan R., and Carol L. Cheatham. "Brain and Behavior Interface: Stress and the developing brain." *Infant Mental Health Journal* 24 (2003): 195–211.

Gutteling, Barbara, Carolina de Weerth, and Jan K. Buitelaar. "Prenatal stress and children's cortisol reaction to the first day of school." *Psychoneuroendocrinology* 30 (2005): 541–49.

Gutteling, Barbara, Carolina de Weerth, Noortje Zandbelt, Eduard J. H. Mulder, Gerard H. A. Visser, and Jan K. Buitelaar. "Does Maternal Prenatal Stress Adversely Affect the Child's Learning and Memory at Age Six?" *Journal of Abnormal Child Psychology* 34 (2006): 787–96.

Hampton, Tracy. "Stress and Memory Loss Link." *Journal of the American Medical Association* 292 (2004): 2963.

Hay, Louise. *You Can Heal Your Life*. Carlsbad, CA: Hay House, 1999.

Henry, Chantal, Mohamed Kabbaj, Herve Simon, Michel Le Moal, and Stefania Maccari. "Prenatal Stress Increases the Hypothalamo-Pituitary-Adrenal Axis Response in Young and Adult Rats." *Journal of Neuroendocrinology* 6 (2006): 341–45.

Hobel, Calvin J., Christine Dunkel-Schetter, Scott C. Roesch, Lony C. Castro, and Chander P. Arora. "Maternal plasma corticotropin-releasing hormone associated with stress at 20 weeks' gestation in pregnancies ending in preterm delivery." *American Journal of Obstetrics and Gynecology* 180 (1999): S257–63.

Hobel, Calvin, J., A. Goldstein, and E. S. Barrett. "Psychosocial stress and pregnancy outcome." *Clinical Obstetrics and Gynecology* 51 (2008): 333–48.

Huizink, Anja C., Eduard J. Mulder, Pascale G. Robles de Medina, Gerard H. A. Visser, and Jan K. Buitelaar. "Is pregnancy anxiety a distinctive syndrome?" *Early Human Development* 79 (2004): 81–91.

Huizink, Anja C., Pascale G. Robles de Medina, Eduard J. H. Mulder, Gerard H. A. Visser, and Jan K. Buitelaar. "Stress during pregnancy is associated with developmental outcome in infancy." *Journal of Child Psychology and Psychiatry* 44 (2003): 810–18.

Karren, Keith. J., Lee Smith, Brent Q. Hafen, and Kathryn J. Frandsen. *Mind/Body Health: The Effects of Attitudes, Emotions, and Relationships*, 4th ed. San Francisco: Benjamin Cummings, 2009.

Khalfa, Stéphanie, Simone Dalla Bella, Mathieu Roy, Isabelle Peretz, and Sonia J. Lupien. "Effects of Relaxing Music on Salivary Cortisol Level after Psychological Stress." *Annals of New York Academy of Science* 999 (2003): 374–76.

Kinney, Dennis K., Kerim M. Munir, David J. Crowley, and Andrea M. Miller. "Prenatal Stress and Risk for Autism." *Neuroscience and Biobehavioral Reviews* 32 (2008): 1519–32.

Kirschbaum, Clemens, and Dirk H. Hellhammer. "The 'Trier Social Stress Test' a tool for investigating psychobiology stress responses in a laboratory setting." *Neuropsychobiology* 28 (1993):
76–81.

Kirschbaum, Clemens, and Dirk H. Hellhammer. "Salivary cortisol
in psychoneuroendocrine research: recent developments and
applications." *Psychoneuroendocrinology* 19 (1994): 313–33.

Klopfenstein, A. "Die Tomatis babies." In Alfred A. Tomatis, ed.
Klangwelt Mutterleib. Munich, Germany: Kösel-Verlag, 1994),
132–56.

Kofman, Ora. "The role of prenatal stress in the etiology of
developmental behavioural disorders." *Neuroscience and
Biobehavioral Reviews* 26 (2002): 457–70.

Laplante, David P., Ronald G. Barr, Alain Brunet, Guillaume
Galbaud du Fort, Michael L. Meaney, Jean-Francois Saucier,
Philip R. Zelazo, and Suzanne King. "Stress during pregnancy
affects general intellectual and language functioning in human
toddlers." *Pediatric Research* 56 (2004): 400–10.

Laplante, David P., Alain Brunet, Norbert Schmitz, Antonio
Ciampi, and Suzanne King. "Project Ice Storm: prenatal
maternal stress affects cognitive and linguistic functioning
in 5½-year-old children." *Journal of the American Academy of
Child and Adolescent Psychiatry* 47 (2008): 1063–72.

Lemaire, Valerie, Muriel Koehl, Michael Le Moal, and Djoher N.
Abrous. "Prenatal stress produces learning deficits associated
with an inhibition of neurogenesis in the hippocampus."
*Proceedings of the National Academy of Sciences of the United
States of America* 97 (2000): 11032–37.

LeWinn, Kaja Z., Laura R. Stroud, Beth E. Molnar, James H.
Ware, Karestan C. Koenen, and Stephen L. Buka. "Elevated
maternal cortisol levels during pregnancy are associated with
reduced childhood IQ." *International Journal of Epidemiology*
10 (2009): 1–11.

Linnet, Karen M., Soren Dalsgaard, Carsten Obel, Kirsten Wisborg,
Tine Brink Hendriksen, Alina Rodriguez, Arto Kotimaa,
Irma Moilanen, Per Hove Thomsen, Jorn Olsen, and Marjo-
Riitta Jarvelin. "Maternal Lifestyle Factors in Pregnancy Risk

of Attention Deficit Hyperactivity Disorder and Associated Behaviors: Review of the Current Evidence." *American Journal of Psychiatry* 160 (2003): 1028–40.

Lupien, Sonja J., Mony de Leon, Susan de Santi, Antonio Convit, Chaim Tarshish, N. P. V. Nair, Mika Thakur, Bruce S. McEwen, Richard L. Hauger, and Michael J. Meaney. "Cortisol levels during human aging predict hippocampal atrophy and memory deficits." *Nature Neuroscience* 1 (1998): 69–73.

Madaule, Paul. *When Listening Comes Alive: A Guide to Effective Learning and Communication*, 2nd ed. Ontario, Canada: Moulin Publishing, 1997.

McArdle, William D., Frank I. Katch and Victor L. Katch. *Exercise Physiology: Energy, Nutrition, and Human Physiology*, 6th ed. New York: Lippincott Williams and Wilkins, 2006, 270.

Mandell, David S., William W. Thompson, Eric S. Weintraub, Frank DeStefano, and Michael B. Blank, "Trends in diagnostic rates for autism and ADHD at hospital discharge in the context of other psychiatric diagnoses." *Psychiatric Services* 56 (2005): 56–62.

Monk, Catherine, Michael Myers, Richard Sloan, Lauren Ellman, and William Fifer. "Effects of Women's Stress-Elicited Physiological Activity and Chronic Anxiety on Fetal Heart Rate." *Journal of Developmental and Behavioral Pediatrics* 24 (2003): 32–38.

Monk, Catherine, Richard P. Sloan, Michael Myers, Lauren M. Ellman, Elizabeth Werner, Jiyeon Jeon, Felice Tager, and William P. Fifer. "Fetal heart rate reactivity differs by women's psychiatric status: An early marker for developmental risk." *Journal of the American Academy of Child and Adolescent Psychiatry* 43 (2004): 283–90.

Mulder, Eduard J. H., Pascalle Robles de Medina, Anja Huizink, Bea R. H. Van den Bergh, Jan K. Buitelaar, and Gerard Visser. "Prenatal Maternal Stress: effects on pregnancy and the (unborn) child." *Early Human Development* 70 (2002), 3–14.

Murkoff, Heidi, and Sharon Mazel. *What to Expect When You're Expecting*, 4th ed. New York: Workman Publishing Co., 2008.

Nepomnaschy, Pablo A., Kathleen B. Welch, Daniel S. McConnell, Bobbi S. Low, Beverly I. Strassmann, and Barry G. England. "Cortisol levels and very early pregnancy loss in humans. *Proceedings of the National Academy of Sciences of the United States of America* 103 (2006): 3938–42.

O'Connor, Thomas. G., Yoav Ben-Shlomo, Jonathan Heron, Jean Golding, Diana Adams, and Vivette Glover. "Prenatal Anxiety Predicts Individual Differences in Cortisol in Pre-Adolescent Children." Biological Psychiatry 58 (2005): 211–17.

O'Connor, Thomas G., Jonathan Heron, Vivette Glover, and ALSPAC Study Team. "Antenatal anxiety predicts child behavioral/emotional problems independently of postnatal depression." *Journal of the American Academy of Child and Adolescent Psychiatry* 41 (2002): 1470–77.

O'Connor, Thomas G., Jonathan Heron, Jean Golding, Michael Beveridge, and Vivette Glover. "Maternal antenatal anxiety and children's behavioural/emotional problems at 4 years. Report from the Avon Longitudinal Study of Parents and Children." *British Journal of Psychiatry* 180 (2002): 502–8.

O'Connor, Thomas G., Jonathan Heron, Jean Golding, Vivette Glover, and ALSPAC Study Team. "Maternal antenatal anxiety and behavioural/emotional problems in children: a test of a programming hypothesis." *Journal of Child Psychology and Psychiatry* 44 (2003): 1025–36.

Oates, Margaret R. "Adverse effects of maternal antenatal anxiety on children: causal effect or developmental continuum?" *British Journal of Psychiatry* 180 (2002): 478–79.

Paul, Annie M. Origins: *How the Nine Months Before Birth Shape the Rest of Our Lives*. New York: Free Press, 2010.

Pearce, Joseph Chilton. *The Magical Child*. New York: Plume Books, 1977.

Pearce, Joseph Chilton. *Evolution's End: Claiming the Potential of Our Intelligence*. New York: Harper Collins, 1992.

Porges, Stephen W., W. R. Arnold, and E. J. Forbes. "Heart rate variability: an index of attentional responsivity in newborns." *Developmental Psychology* 8 (1973): 85–92.

Relier, Jean-Pierre. "Influence of Maternal Stress on Fetal Behavior and Brain Development." *Biology of the Neonate* 79 (2001): 167–71.

Sacks, Oliver. *Musicophilia: Tales of Music and the Brain.* New York: Vintage Books, 2007.

Schwartz, Fred J. "Perinatal Stress Reduction, Music and Medical Cost Savings." *Journal of Prenatal and Perinatal Psychology and Health* 12 (1997), 19 ff. http://birthpsychology.com/journal-article/perinatal-stress-reduction-music-and-medical-cost-savings.

Scheider, Mary L., and Colleen F. Moore. "The impact of prenatal stress, fetal alcohol exposure, or both on development: perspectives from a primate model." *Psychoneuroendocrinology* 27 (2002): 285–98.

Schneider, Mary L., and Christopher L. Coe. "Repeated Social Stress during Pregnancy Impairs Neuromotor Development of the Primate Infant." *Journal of Developmental and Behavioral Pediatrics* 14 (1993): 81–87.

Scott, Elaine M., H. H. G. McGarrigle, and Gillian C. L. Lachelin. "The Increase in Plasma and Saliva Cortisol Levels in Pregnancy is not due to the Increase in Corticosteroid-Binding Globulin Levels." *Journal of Clinical Endocrinology and Metabolism* 71 (1990): 639–44.

Selye, Hans. "Stress and disease." *Science* 122 (1955): 625–31.

Shonkoff, Jack P.; Andrew S. Garner; and the Committee on Psychosocial Aspects of Child and Family Health; Committee on Early Childhood, Adoptions, and Dependent Care; and Section on Developmental and Behavioral Pediatrics. "The Lifelong Effects of Early Childhood Adversity and Toxic Stress." *Pediatrics* 129 (2012): e232–46.

Sollier, Pierre. *Listening for Wellness: An Introduction to the Tomatis Method.* Walnut Creek, CA: The Mozart Center Press, 2005.

Teixeira, Jeronima M., Nicholas M. Fisk, and Vivette Glover. "Association between maternal anxiety in pregnancy and increased uterine artery resistance index: cohort based study." *British Medical Journal* 318 (1999): 153–57.

Thompson, Billie. M., and Susan R. Andrews. "The Emerging Field of Sound Training: Technologies and Methods." *IEEE Engineering in Medicine and Biology. The Institute of Electrical and Electronics Engineers* 18 (1999): 89–96.

Thompson, Billie. M., and Susan R. Andrews. "An Historical Commentary on the Physiological Effects of Music: Tomatis, Mozart and Neuropsychology." *Integrative Physiological and Behavioral Science* 35 (2000): 174–88.

Thompson, William R. "Influence of prenatal maternal anxiety on emotionality in young rats." *Science* 125 (1957): 698–99.

Tomatis, Alfred A. *La Nuit Uterine*. Paris: Edition Stock, 1980.

Tomatis, Alfred A. "Ontogenesis of the faculty of listening." In T. R. Verny, ed. *Pre- and Perinatal Psychology: An Introduction*. New York: Human Sciences Press, 1987, 23–35.

Trenerry, M. R., B. Crosson, J. DeBoe, and W. Leber. *The Stroop Neuropsychological Screening Test*. Odessa, FL: Psychological Assessment Resources, 1989.

Vallée, Monique, Willy Mayo, Francoise Dellu, Michel Le Moal, Hervé Simon, and Stefania Maccari. "Prenatal Stress Induces High Anxiety and Postnatal Handling Induces Low Anxiety in Adult Offspring: Correlation with Stress-Induced Corticosterone Secretion." *The Journal of Neuroscience* 17 (1997): 2626–36.

Van den Bergh, Bea R. H., and Alfons Marcoen. "High Antenatal Maternal Anxiety Is Related to ADHD Symptoms, Externalizing Problems, and Anxiety in 8- and 9-year-olds." *Child Development* 75 (2004): 1085–97.

Van den Bergh, Bea R. H., Ben Van Calster, Tim Smits, Sabine Van Huffel, and Lieven Lagae. "Antenatal Maternal Anxiety is Related to HPA-Axis Dysregulation and Self-Reported Depressive Symptoms in Adolescence: A Prospective Study on the Fetal Origins of Depressed Mood." *Neuropsychopharmacology* 33 (2008): 536–45.

van der Wal, Marcel F., Manon van Eijsden, and G. J. Bonsel. "Stress and emotional problems during pregnancy and excessive infant crying." *Journal of Developmental and Behavioral Pediatrics* 28 (2007): 431–37.

van Os, Jim, and Jean-Paul Selten. "Prenatal exposure to maternal stress and subsequent schizophrenia. The May 1940 invasion of The Netherlands." *British Journal of Psychiatry: The Journal of Mental Health* 172 (1998): 324–26.

Wadhwa, Pathik. D., C. A. Sandman, M. Porto, Christine Dunkel-Schetter, and T. J. Garite. "The association between prenatal stress and infant birth weight and gestational age at birth: a prospective investigation." *American Journal of Obstetrics and Gynecology* 169 (1993): 858–65.

Wakschlag, Lauren S., Benjamin B. Lahey, Rolf Loeber, Stephanie M. Green, Rachel A. Gordon, and Bennett L. Leventhal. "Maternal Smoking During Pregnancy and the Risk of Conduct Disorder in Boys." *Archives General Psychiatry* 54 (1997): 670–76.

Walkup, John T., Anne Marie Albano, John Piacentini, Boris Birmaher, Scott N. Compton, Joel T. Sherrill, Golda S. Ginsburg, Moira A. Rynn, James McCracken, Bruce Waslick, Satish Iyengar, John S. March, and Philip C. Kendall. "Cognitive Behavioral Therapy, Sertraline, or a Combination in Childhood Anxiety." *New England Journal of Medicine* 359 (2008): 2753–66.

Ward, A. J. "A comparison and analysis of the presence of family problems during pregnancy of mothers of 'autistic' children and mothers of normal children." *Child Psychiatry and Human Development* 20 (1990): 279–88.

Weinstock, Marta. "Does prenatal stress impair coping and regulation of hypothalamic-pituitary-adrenal axis?" *Neuroscience and Biobehavioral Review* 21 (1997): 1–10.

Wood, Jeffrey J., Bryce D. McLeod, Marian Sigman, Wei-Chin Hwang, and Brian C. Chu. "Parenting and childhood anxiety: theory, empirical endings, and future directions." *Journal of Child Psychology* 44 (2003): 134–51.

Wright, Rosalind J., Cynthia M. Visness, Agustin Calatroni, Mitchell H. Grayson, Diane R. Gold, Megan T. Sandel, Aviva Lee-Parritz, Robert A. Wood, Meyer Kattan, Gordon R. Bloomberg, Melissa Burger, Alkis Togias, Frank R. Witter, Rhoda S. Sperling, Yoel Sadovsky, and James E. Gern. "Prenatal Maternal Stress and Cord Blood Innate and Adaptive Cytokine Responses in an Inner-City Cohort." *American Journal of Respiratory and Critical Care Medicine* 182 (2010): 25–33.

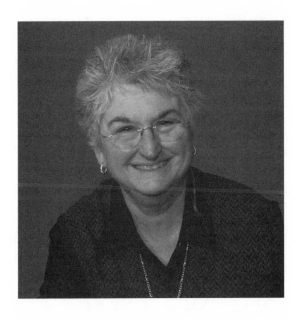

DR. SUSAN ANDREWS is a clinical neuropsychologist whose career has been dedicated to assisting children and their parents improve their quality of life. She helped design Head Start, has been on the staff of several hospital rehabilitation units, and works with children and adults who have suffered traumatic brain injury or have developmental problems, such as language delays, ADD/ADHD, anxiety, and autism. Susan Andrews is also engaged in research at LSU Medical School on traumatic brain injury and anxiety. She lives in the New Orleans area and in Boulder, Colorado. For more resources to help manage stress during pregnancy, including copies of the Stress Solutions worksheets in this book and a community space for sharing your resources and experiences, visit www.StressSolutionsForPregnantMoms.com.